A Compendium of Chronic Obstructive Pulmonary Disease

Edited by Kian Chung Ong

Published in London, United Kingdom

A Compendium of Chronic Obstructive Pulmonary Disease
http://dx.doi.org/10.5772/intechopen.102180
Edited by Kian Chung Ong

Contributors
Buntarika Chatreewatanakul, Biruk Getahun, Abebe Ayalew Bekel, Xiang He, Lei Zhang, Jiliu Liu, Yi Zhang, Xiaohui Zuo, Guoping Li, Aigoul Zinnatullina, Rustem Khamitov, Takashi Sato, Takeshi Shimosato, Hiroaki Kume, Ryuki Yamada, Yuki Sato, Christian Peiser, Kian Chung Ong

First published in London, United Kingdom, 2023 by IntechOpen
IntechOpen is the global imprint of INTECHOPEN LIMITED, registered in England and Wales, registration number: 11086078, 5 Princes Gate Court, London, SW7 2QJ, United Kingdom

British Library Cataloguing-in-Publication Data
A catalogue record for this book is available from the British Library

Additional hard and PDF copies can be obtained from orders@intechopen.com

A Compendium of Chronic Obstructive Pulmonary Disease
Edited by Kian Chung Ong
p. cm.
Print ISBN 978-1-80356-767-9
Online ISBN 978-1-80356-768-6
eBook (PDF) ISBN 978-1-80356-769-3

Meet the editor

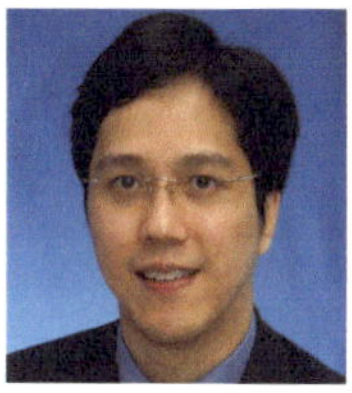

Dr. Kian Chung Ong is a specialist in respiratory and intensive care medicine who completed his advanced training at the Singapore General Hospital in 1998. He works in a private specialist practice at the Chestmed Clinic, Mount Elizabeth Medical Centre, Singapore. Among Dr. Ong's clinical achievements is the establishment of treatment modalities such as pulmonary rehabilitation, non-invasive ventilation, and hospital-at-home programmes for patients with chronic respiratory disorders in Singapore. His research interests include sleep-related breathing disorders, pulmonary function and exercise testing, and chronic obstructive pulmonary disease. Dr. Ong is the president of the Chronic Obstructive Pulmonary Disease Association in Singapore and is a member of the Global Initiative for Chronic Obstructive Lung Disease (GOLD) Assembly.

Contents

Preface

A disorder as common and complex as a chronic obstructive pulmonary disease (COPD) requires frequent updates to our knowledge base. This book provides such a platform. It is written by experts in the field who share a common desire to provide contemporary and critical knowledge on COPD.

Chapter 1 describes the evolution of our knowledge of COPD through the decades while emphasizing the need for contextualization to successfully integrate research with practice today. Chapter 2 is a state-of-the-art compilation of all that is essential and evolving in COPD. It discusses "hot topics" in COPD, a "multi-aspect" exploration of COPD. The reader will certainly appreciate the discursive journey into the contemporary conceptions of COPD, moving from pathogenesis to treatment. Chapter 3 is an excellent summary of recent scientific findings on inflammation in COPD and is testimony to the ardor of the author in filtering through the vast amount of basic research in this area to present the data systematically, succinctly, and concisely.

Chapters 4 and 5 offer a change in emphasis, form, and content. They present the results of two retrospective single-center observational studies describing the risk factors associated with repeated hospitalization for exacerbation of COPD in different cultures and locales. These series contribute to the existing literature by their description of local statistics while highlighting the need for effective strategies to reduce the heavy burden of exacerbation of COPD throughout the world. The reader is thus reminded of the need to consider local and global factors when implementing strategies to reduce COPD exacerbation.

Chapter 6 discusses therapeutics for COPD, specifically pulmonary rehabilitation. It elucidates the benefits and practical aspects of a comprehensive pulmonary rehabilitation program for patients with COPD. Chapter 7 delves further into specific therapeutics and precision medicine, highlighting the role of phenotypes and endotypes in directing inhaled therapy in COPD. Finally, Chapter 8 points toward the future. Under careful consideration is the intriguing plausibility of intratracheal administration of biologically active molecules as a delivery tool or as therapeutic agents for the treatment and prevention of COPD.

I hope that this publication will prove useful for all who share an academic interest in progressive scientific research and best practices in COPD. Last and not least,

I would like to express my appreciation to the chapter authors as well as Author Service Manager Martina Scerbe at IntechOpen for her contribution and assistance in making this publication a reality.

Kian Chung Ong
Mount Elizabeth Medical Centre,
Singapore

Chapter 1

Introductory Chapter: Contextualizing Chronic Obstructive Pulmonary Disease

Kian Chung Ong

1. Introduction

Chronic Obstructive Pulmonary Disease (COPD) afflicts more than 390 million people globally [1] and is the third leading cause of death worldwide [2]. COPD is also a heterogeneous and complex malady, varying in severity and clinical presentation. The commonness and the complexity of this disorder require contextualization in balancing global scientific development with the local milieu, and the general aspects of the disease with particular subject characteristics.

2. Evaluating COPD in different contexts

Perhaps more so than other common respiratory disorders such as bronchial asthma, the construal of COPD varies according to demographic, cultural, socio-economic, geographical, and even political contexts. Patients' anamnesis and conceptions of the illness not only vary across the world but also according to the chronological period that the disease is diagnosed. Change in nomenclature has contributed somewhat to the latter. Nowadays, terms like "chronic bronchitis" and "emphysema" are less often used in clinical diagnosis, and in their place, the acronym COPD has become widely accepted across the globe by laymen and professionals. The benefit of standard terminology is not solely titular since the definition of the disease can only be agreed upon once everyone has accepted what it should be called, at least in clinical practice. For this, we are heavily indebted to the unifying work developed and continually updated by the Global Initiative for Chronic Obstructive Lung Disease (GOLD) [3] in enabling clinicians and researchers to figuratively speak the same language. Some readers may recall an epoch when COPD was confusingly construed as overlapping conditions of chronic bronchitis, emphysema, and asthma within the confines of chronic airflow limitation. In appreciation of GOLD, standard definitions of COPD have been refined and gained widespread acceptance, thus fostering mutual understanding and expedient communication within the medical community.

Nonetheless, such universality in evaluating COPD tends to mask the particularity of COPD as it presents in various contexts. The term COPD confers varying connotations among diverse individuals and people groups. For instance, diagnosis of COPD will likely evoke more unease among people where the disease is less common than in populations with shared predisposing factors leading to a high prevalence of the disease. Contrariwise, detecting COPD in younger patients and non-smoking women may prove challenging for a disease oft erroneously thought to be confined to older smoking men. A diagnosis of COPD made a decade or two ago does not conjure up the same notions compared to one recently established, as the rapid rate of advancement in medical knowledge may have a consequent impact on the minds of both the patient and the clinician. Two score and more years ago, diagnosis of the disease was often met with nihilism, as physicians had little to offer and diagnoses were delayed with scant attention paid to the early stages of COPD. Not much was known about the natural progression of the disease, save for a greater rate of decline in lung function among susceptible smokers compared to healthy adults. Currently, we know that that simplistic paradigm requires a reformation to accommodate multifactorial disease progression, with myriad contributory factors that may be present earlier in life, some even in childhood or *in utero* [4]. This paradigm shift goes some way toward answering the age-old question of why some smokers develop COPD but not others. With such advancement in knowledge, the stigma of COPD as a self-afflicted smoker's disease should also be done away with. In today's context, a diagnosis of COPD should no longer convey a sense of shame for the patient nor an attitude of sanctimony among others.

3. Confronting COPD within different contexts

The age of nihilism should also give way to a future of hope. Historical phenomena such as the stigmatization of smokers who develop COPD and denial of treatment options for those with the severe disease remain significant only as they are related to the responsibility of the present and the promises of the future. An appreciation of different contexts in the clinical presentation of COPD calls for earlier means of diagnosing COPD in an individual patient's lifetime, or at least the ability to predict which individuals are susceptible to COPD. From the newer theoretical understanding of the development of COPD also emanates anticipation of better preventive strategies in the future [4, 5].

In treating COPD, contextualization is crucial. Global guidelines formulated using evidence derived from restricted clinical trial formats are unlikely to be fully relevant to every clinical context in the real world. Clinicians in low-resource countries may be quite adept at managing COPD without the standard spirometry and other tests to rule out differential diagnoses as recommended by global practice guidelines. Recent developments in genomics, phenotyping, endotyping, and identifying treatable traits for the *telos* of personalized medicine may be impracticable in certain settings. Here again is where the universality of COPD, in that it is such a prevalent disease, must be balanced with the particularity of managing COPD within different contexts. Precision medicine does not always entail the use of proteomics and biomarkers, important as they are for the understanding and treatment of the disease, to guide therapeutic decisions. Neither does personalizing medicine mean forsaking the norm or whatever works for the whole, in favor of the quixotic or specific. More empirically, individualizing treatment requires reasoning and adaptation. When confronting COPD in extensive contexts, the clinician must be willing to apply powers of observation and reasoning: *deduction* (what works for the whole or in principle, should work for the individual), *induction* (observe what works for an individual to form a general conclusion), as well as *abduction* (to infer based on observation and assumption).

Additionally, the clinician must be willing to adapt to different or changing contexts when confronting COPD. This is an especially essential trait in an era of scientific progress vitiated by disruptions brought about by the current pandemic. The rapid espousal and widespread use of telehealth and remote monitoring to overcome the physical restrictions due to the pandemic are positive demonstrations of adaptive contextualization of therapeutics in COPD.

In sum, contextualization is important for both evaluating and managing the nuances of this common and complex disorder. Patient and physician education, acceptance and usage of evidence-based guidelines, and therapeutic evolution all require careful contextualization for salubrious practical implementation.

Author details

Kian Chung Ong
Mount Elizabeth Medical Centre, Singapore

*Address all correspondence to: dr@chestmed.com.sg

References

[1] Adeloye D, Song P, Zhu Y, Campbell H, Sheikh A, Rudan I, et al. Global, regional, and national prevalence of, and risk factors for, chronic obstructive pulmonary disease (COPD) in 2019: A systematic review and modelling analysis. The Lancet Respiratory Medicine. 2022;**10**:447-458

[2] Chronic obstructive pulmonary disease (COPD). Available from: https://www.who.int/news-room/fact-sheets/detail/chronic-obstructive-pulmonary-disease-(copd) [Accessed: December 2022]

[3] GOLD 2023 Report. Available from: https://goldcopd.org/2023-gold-report-2/ [Accessed: December 2022]

[4] Lange P, Celli B, Agustí A, Boje Jensen G, Divo M, Faner R, et al. Lung-function trajectories leading to chronic obstructive pulmonary disease. The New England Journal of Medicine. 2015;**373**:111-122

[5] Krishnan JK, Martinez FJ. Lung function trajectories and chronic obstructive pulmonary disease: Current understanding and knowledge gaps. Current Opinion in Pulmonary Medicine. 2018;**24**:124-129

Chapter 2

Exploration of Multi-Aspect Development of Chronic Obstructive Pulmonary Disease Pathogenesis, Diagnosis, and Treatment Management

Lei Zhang, Xiang He, Jiliu Liu, Yi Zhang, Xiaohui Zuo and Guoping Li

Abstract

Chronic obstructive pulmonary disease (COPD) is a common, preventable, and treatable chronic respiratory disease, which is characterized by persistent airflow limitation and respiratory symptoms. Pathological changes are mainly airway and/or alveolar structural abnormalities. Numerous factors, such as exposure to harmful particles or gases, genetic susceptibility, abnormal inflammatory responses, and abnormal lung development, are involved in the pathogenesis of COPD, those which determine the heterogeneity of COPD. Individuals show different pathophysiological changes, different disease evolution rules, and different clinical manifestations due to different etiologies, different susceptibility genes, and different chronic processes of "injury-inflammation-repair." Therefore, disease managers need to conduct a multifaceted assessment of the whole body and the local area from the individual characteristics of COPD. With the sustained advancement of new technologies, from multiple perspectives, including genomics, exposomes, transcriptomics, mechanisms related to inflammation and immune regulation, microbiota, metabolomics, imaging features and radiomics, and the interaction of lungs and systemic organs to further explore the law of the occurrence and development of COPD, and finally, form an optimized prevention and treatment strategy. On the basis of thorough exploration, a COPD evaluation system that can meet clinical needs will be finally formed, so as to formulate scientific and effective individualized management strategies.

Keywords: chronic obstructive pulmonary disease, COPD pathogenesis, COPD diagnosis, COPD management

1. Introduction

Chronic obstructive pulmonary disease (COPD) is a common, preventable, and treatable disease worldwide, characterized by persistent airflow limitation and associated respiratory symptoms. Its pathological features are mainly chronic inflammatory changes in airway, lung parenchyma, and pulmonary vessels, which are usually associated with exposure to harmful particles and gases. Many factors, such as genetic susceptibility, abnormal inflammatory response, and abnormal lung development, are involved in the pathogenesis. In 2020, there were about 550 million (about 7.4%) COPD patients in the world, with the highest proportion of patients with COPD in Oceania (about 10.9%) and the lowest in Africa (about 5.4%) [1]. It mainly affects the population over 40 years old. Men and women are at equal risk. In 1990, COPD caused appropriate 2.4 million deaths. Until 2019, the global deaths rose to 3.23 million. About 80% of the deaths occurred in low- and middle-income countries, on the one hand, due to the high prevalence of smoking. On the other hand, it is difficult for the public and medical workers to obtain information on diagnosis and treatment management in terms of the low coverage of COPD diagnosis (69.8% in low- and middle-income countries, 98.1% in high-income countries) [2]. With the increasing smoking rate in developing countries and the aging population in high-income countries, the latest data of the World Health Organization show that the prevalence of COPD will continue to rise in the next 40 years with more than 5.4 million deaths from COPD and its related diseases annually by 2060. COPD has become an important public health problem in the world because of its high incidence, high mortality, and social and economic burden. Advances in pulmonary imaging have enabled more detailed understandings of airway and parenchymal abnormalities, and new endoscopic interventions are playing an increasingly important role in the management of advanced emphysema. At present, there is still no etiology-specific treatment for emphysema other than the addition of alpha 1 antitrypsin in patients with emphysema associated with alpha 1 antitrypsin deficiency. Further prospective studies could help clarify the role of inhaled corticosteroids in combination with dual bronchodilator therapy in the prevention of exacerbations. Compared with asthma, there is little hope for developing COPD-specific biotherapies. However, we still cannot give up investigation of COPD pathogenesis and developing scientific prevention and management methods. Therefore, this chapter focuses on the pathogenesis of COPD and the latest research advances in treatment and management of COPD.

2. Research advances in the pathogenesis of COPD

Clinical guidelines issued by the Global Initiative for Chronic Obstructive Lung Disease (GOLD) tend to simplify the definition of COPD. COPD is actually a heterogeneous and complex disease. Smoking is globally recognized as the most important risk factor for COPD. But data from population-based studies show that only half of COPD cases are caused by smoking. Reports from South Africa, China, and South Korea indicate that the proportion of non-smoking COPD in men and women was different, and the morbidity of non-smoking COPD in women was more than 50%, suggesting that it may be related to household smoke exposure. COPD caused by exposure to biomass fuels is quite different from smoking-induced COPD in terms of phenotype, morbidity, and disease progression. Tuberculosis infection, occupational exposure, and frequent infections in children are also considered as major risks for the development of COPD. Agriculture is also a risk factor for COPD, where pesticide exposure is associated with accelerated decline in lung function, with a reduction of 6.9 ml per year in forced expiratory volume in 1 second (FEV 1). In addition to environmental exposure, genetic risk factors are increasingly associated with the development of nicotine addiction, chronic bronchitis, loss of lung function, and early lung development.

Unregulated inflammation, oxidative/antioxidant imbalance, proteolytic/anti-proteolytic imbalance, and imbalance of cell damage/repair are recognized mechanisms. At the same time, microbiota bias, air-pollutant-related damage, and autoimmune processes in lung tissue are all underlying pathogenesis of COPD. Epigenetic regulation has also been implicated in the pathogenesis of COPD.

2.1 Inflammatory mechanism

The pathological changes of COPD are characterized by chronic inflammation of airway, lung parenchyma, and pulmonary vessels. When the body inhales harmful particles and gases, it can cause a variety of inflammatory cells to participate in the release of a variety of inflammatory mediators, leading to irreversible lung damage. Damage to airway epithelial cells triggers a nonspecific inflammatory response through the release of endogenous intracellular molecules or risk-associated molecular patterns. These signals are recognized by pattern recognition receptors such as Toll-like receptors 4 and 2 on epithelial cells, resulting in the release of cytokines, such as TNF-α, IL-1β, granulocyte-macrophage colony-stimulating factor (GM-CSF), transforming growth factor (TGF) -β1, MCP-1, LTB 4, and IL-8. Inflammatory cells such as macrophages, neutrophils, eosinophils, and dendritic cells are recruited to sites of inflammation to form innate immune responses, while Th1, Th17, and ILC3 lymphocytes constitute acquired immunity. At the same time, activated inflammatory cells release a variety of inflammatory mediators. The mediators act on airway epithelial cells, which in turn promote epithelial cell damage. In patients with COPD, tissue damage by inflammation is uninterrupted, and the inflammatory response persists even after smoking cessation. In the case of chronic bronchitis, prolonged exposure to risk factors leads to mucosal and glandular inflammation, increased mucus secretion and epithelial cell proliferation, and altered tissue repair of the small airways.

Circulating blood cells, including neutrophils, and inflammatory cells in the lungs have long been implicated as players in smoking-induced tissue damage. Neutrophils in the sputum and bronchoalveolar lavage fluid (BALF) of patients with COPD are found to rapidly appear at sites of inflammation in response to interleukin (IL) -8, and neutrophil numbers increase with interleukin (IL) -6. A variety of other chemokines can induce neutrophil migration, including chemokines CXC motif ligand 2 (CXCL2), leukotriene B4 (LTB4), and formyl-met-leuphe (fMLP), which are produced by the body's own immune cells and diseased tissue cells and are related to host-microbe interactions. Alpha-1-antitrypsin (AAT) is the major anti-protease, which is also a candidate chemokine for neutrophils. Neutrophils are major destroyers of the elastic matrix of the alveoli. By secreting proteases and small cationic peptides, neutrophils are able to attack invading bacteria, viruses, pollutants, and in some autoimmune situations, their own tissues. Under the influence of environmental pollution (including cigarette smoke), enzymes and peptides released by neutrophils are able to cut collagen into pieces, thereby activating inflammatory cells and driving further chronic inflammation.

Circulating progenitors of pulmonary macrophages are originated from mononuclear cells in peripheral blood. When local inflammation occurs in the airways, monocytes migrate from the circulatory system to the lung tissue and differentiate into interstitial and alveolar macrophages. Pulmonary macrophages coexist with emphysematous areas and increase in number in the airways, lung parenchyma, BALF, and sputum of patients. The number of macrophages in the airways is positively correlated with the severity of COPD. Macrophages can be activated by cigarette smoke extracts to release inflammatory mediators including tumor necrosis factor (TNF) -a, interleukin-8, other chemokines such as CXCL9, CXCL10, and CXCL11, monocyte chemotactic peptide (MCP) -1, LTb4, and reactive oxygen species. In addition, alveolar macrophages also secrete elastase including MMP-2, MMP-9, MMP-12, cathepsins K, L, and S, and neutrophil elastase extracted from neutrophils. Inflammatory proteins that are upregulated in macrophages during acute exacerbations of COPD are regulated by transcription factors such as nuclear factor-κB (NF-κB), activator protein-1, and tyrosine kinase c-Src.

T lymphocytes are present in the entire human organism including the epithelial surface of lung and mediate host defense. Human lungs are rich in resident T cells (more than 10 billion). Th1-type cells are involved in a sustained autoimmune response with interferon gamma as the primary cytokine and lead to exaggerated pro-inflammatory responses that result in uncontrolled tissue damage. Emphysema is generally considered to be a Th1 disease. Studies have shown that the development of emphysema may be mediated by T lymphocytes, and all T cell phenotypes are increased in smokers with COPD. Although neutrophils are the predominant cells in the lung parenchyma of non-COPD smokers, there is an increase in T cells (CD3 and CD8), primarily CD8 cytotoxic T cells, with evidence of emphysema. Apoptosis may be one of the mechanisms of pulmonary emphysema. In emphysema, CD8 T-cell numbers are correlated with the severity of tissue destruction, and their accumulation continues even after smoking cessation. In addition, the number of T cells was correlated with smoking history. In conclusion, the different interrelationships between T cell subtypes in COPD may be important for the progression of inflammation.

Airway eosinophilia and Th2-type inflammation are associated with allergic airway diseases such as asthma. However, recent studies have reported that 20–40% of COPD patients exhibit stable sputum eosinophilia. The SPIROMICS (SubPopulations and InteRmediate Outcome Measures In COPD Study) cohort has found that stable sputum eosinophilia is related to an increased frequency of disease exacerbations. In the meantime, high blood eosinophil levels at steady state predict a better therapeutic response to inhaled corticosteroids, which may be used to guide treatment. Although stable sputum and blood eosinophilia would be regarded as biomarkers of disease and steroid responsiveness, further work is needed to assess the importance of increased Th2 inflammation during COPD exacerbations.

2.2 Oxidative stress/antioxidant imbalance

ROS are oxygen-rich unstable molecules that can be either donors or acceptors of free electrons. Intracellular ROS can induce functional and structural changes in cells. The intracellular redox state is determined by the oxidant load in the respirable air and the pooling capacity of the lung protective mechanisms to absorb oxidants. Alveolar lining fluid, alveolar epithelial cells, local macrophages, and lung fibroblasts are all major targets of ROS. They can also be a secondary source of ROS. It showed that most cell types induce ROS production, and all lung cells may be involved in the redox state transition of COPD. The body keeps a dynamic balance between oxidation and antioxidation in normal condition. However, under pathological conditions, the imbalance between oxidation and antioxidation leads to oxidative stress, lipid peroxidation, protein modification, DNA damage, and activation of pro-inflammatory factors such as transcription factors NF-κB, which initiate inflammatory response and further promote oxidative stress. At the same time, the increase of oxidant can initiate the expression of antioxidant and anti-inflammatory genes through activation of nuclear factor E2-related factor (Nrf2). Therefore, antioxidant therapy may be effective in controlling and alleviating the symptoms and disease progression of COPD. Both outdoor environmental smoke and indoor airs are sources of environmental ROS. For example, laser printers can significantly increase indoor air pollution from ozone and volatile organic compounds (VOCs), and appropriate filters may reduce this pollution. In addition, office buildings are carpeted with pesticides, and the use of caustic cleaning products can produce large amounts of inhalable chemicals and particles. Aerosol spray products, air fresheners, chlorine bleaches, cleaners, dry cleaning chemicals, and furniture and floor polishes may release VOCs and other toxic substances. Therefore, it is necessary to install proper ventilation and ventilation devices.

2.3 Imbalance of protease and anti-protease

Proteolytic enzymes have damaging and destructive effects on tissues, while anti-protease inhibits the activity of elastase. Imbalanced proteolysis is a plausible mechanism to explain the long-term persistence of emphysema. This theory partly explains the development of COPD. Proteolytic enzymes in healthy human lungs are resisted by anti-proteases. When exposed to cigarette smoke, this balance is broken and tends to proteolysis. Cigarette smoke or irritants derived from polluted air recruit inflammatory cells to produce protease 3, cathepsins L and S, MMP-2, MMP-9, and MMP-12, which are secreted primarily by neutrophils and macrophages. The anti-proteolytic barrier is composed of AAT, secretory leukocyte protease inhibitor, and tissue inhibitors of MMPs (TIMPs). Various modified forms of AAT (oxidized, aggregated, cleaved, nitrated, and citrullinated) have been implicated in inflammatory lung tissue destruction, of which proteolysis and ROS attack are major processes. Deficiency of α1-antiprotease causes an imbalance between protease and anti-protease, resulting in emphysema. In addition to proteolytic enzymes and inhibitory substances secreted by host inflammatory cells, bacterial enzymes and inhibitors should also be considered. In lung fibroblasts, elastase released by *Pseudomonas aeruginosa* activates the epidermal growth factor receptor (EGFR)/extracellular signal-regulated kinase (ERK) signaling pathway to promote IL-8 production by upregulating NF-κB. Besides proteases from neutrophils and macrophages, matrix metalloproteinases (MMPs) secreted by structural cells also play important roles in the pathogenesis of COPD. A number of MMPs members have been found to be involved in the process of COPD. Among them, MMP-1 is usually produced by fibroblasts, and MMP-8 is mainly expressed by neutrophils, both of which have collagenase activity and destroy the normal structure of alveolar septa. MMP-9 is produced by macrophages, neutrophils, and epithelial cells, not only to degrade ECM, but also to activate the immune response through the production of N-acetylproline-glycine-proline chemokines. MMPs can degrade almost all components of the extracellular matrix (ECM). ECM is hydrolyzed into peptide fragments that can promote local inflammation, which play a chemotactic role. For example, after MMP-12 degrades elastin, the peptide fragments have chemotactic effects on monocytes and fibroblasts, promote inflammatory responses, and accelerate lung tissue damage. Proteolytic products of ECM may perpetuate inflammation even after smoking cessation. Therefore, the level of elastin degradation products can be used as a good indicator of lung injury. As in COPD patients with α1 antitrypsin deficiency, a known genetic background (endotype) with distinct clinical manifestations (phenotype) of emphysema leads to targeted therapeutic intervention (enhancing α1 antitrypsin). Major advances in lung imaging have paved the way to a new concept of COPD diversity. We need a more detailed understanding of the risk factors that contribute to these different endotypes and phenotypes to better describe therapeutic interventions.

2.4 Cell senescence and apoptosis

Cell senescence is an irreversible cell cycle arrest, which is a normal physiological phenomenon. Normal aging and emphysema share common pathophysiological features including the enlargement of alveolar space and the loss of elastic recoil. The accumulation of senescent cells in the body with aging leading to a senescence-associated secretion phenotype (senescence-related secretory phenotype, SASP) induces a pro-inflammatory state, which plays an important role in various age-related diseases. At present, the mechanisms of cell aging involved in COPD include oxidative stress, telomere shortening, mitochondrial dysfunction, activation of mTOR signal transduction, reduction of antiaging molecules, stem cell failure, and DNA damage repair defects. Cell senescence usually results in reduced proliferation with unchanged metabolic activity. This leads to increase inflammation and reduce cell regeneration, a process that is further accelerated by smoking and oxidative stress. Aging affects lung structures and inflammatory cells, fibroblasts, and progenitor cells, resulting in insufficient repair and regeneration. Defective clearance of apoptotic cells in patients with emphysema contributes to the persistence of pulmonary inflammation and increases the risk of acute exacerbation. It is also one of the important reasons leading to the progressive decline of lung function in patients. Autophagy dysregulation is present in cells from COPD patients as well. Insufficient autophagy results in the accumulation of the contents of damaged cells, causing senescence. In the normal lung, autophagy maintains a balance between organelle and protein production, degradation, and recycling. In COPD lung, chronic imbalance in autophagy leads to increased tissue senescence and insufficient repair.

2.5 Pathogenesis of COPD acute exacerbation

The common symptom of AECOPD is transient dyspnea, sputum suppuration, and increased sputum volume. Mild symptoms also occur, such as nasal obstruction, wheezing, sore throat, cough, fever, chest tightness, fatigue, insomnia, or physical activity limitation. In most cases, exacerbation in inflammatory airway is triggered by infection. Respiratory virus (rhinovirus, influenza virus, RSV, parainfluenza virus, human metapneumovirus, coronavirus, and adenovirus) infection is the main cause. Bacterial infection and environmental factors such as air pollution and ambient temperature also trigger or aggravate acute events. Meanwhile, heart failure, pneumothorax, pulmonary embolism, and anxiety cause acute exacerbation. Rhinoviruses account for 60% of exacerbations, which is the most prevalent predisposing factor. At present, it is believed that the antiviral immunity of COPD patients is impaired after respiratory viral infection, but the specific mechanism of aggravation of the disease is not fully understood. Bacteria are also extremely important in the pathogenesis of COPD exacerbations. Common species include the nontypeable *Haemophilus influenzae*, *Moraxella catarrhalis*, *Streptococcus pneumoniae*, and *Pseudomonas aeruginosa*, with *Mycoplasma pneumoniae* and *Chlamydia pneumoniae* occasionally present. The application of microbiome technology has led to a new understanding of the interaction between the host and millions of microorganisms. 16S ribosomal RNA sequencing reveals that the lungs of healthy people and patients with COPD are colonized by rich, complex bacterial flora. The acute exacerbation is caused by the dysbiosis of preexisting bacteria in the lungs, rather than by the elimination of old species or emergence of new species [3].

AECOPD is also characterized by abnormal airway inflammation. Traditionally, airway eosinophilia and Th2-type inflammation have been associated with allergic airway diseases such as asthma. Recent studies have found that 20–40% of patients with COPD exhibit sputum eosinophilia. The SPIROMICS (SubPopulations and InteRmediate Outcome Measures In COPD Study) cohort has found that sputum eosinophilia in stable state is associated with an increased frequency of COPD exacerbations and deteriorations. In addition, the high level of eosinophil in blood indicates a better therapeutic response to inhaled corticosteroids, which may be used to guide treatment [4]. Although stable sputum and blood eosinophilia are considered as biomarkers of disease outcome and steroid responsiveness, further work is needed to assess the importance of increased Th2 inflammation during COPD exacerbations. In contrast to non-bacterial attacks, bacterial-associated COPD exacerbations result in airway neutrophilia and release of inflammatory mediators including IL-8, leukotriene B4, and TNF-α. Macrophages and T lymphocytes are also involved in the pathogenesis of COPD exacerbation.

These mechanisms mentioned above work together to produce two major pathologies: small airway pressure elevation and emphysema, which cause persistent irreversible airflow limitation. COPD is a chronic disease with high morbidity and mortality, which is a serious threat to human health. Because of its complex etiology and pathogenesis, at present, there are still no effective targeted drugs and treatments. We should further study the cellular and molecular mechanisms in the pathogenesis of COPD in order to detect the disease early and delay disease progression.

2.6 Epigenetic changes in the development of COPD

The imbalanced proteolysis theory is also supported by data from genome-wide association studies (GWAS) and gene expression studies. Recent COPD GWAS studies identified the following genome-wide locus that is strongly associated with the risk and development of COPD, including FAM13a at 4q22, the upstream enhancer of HHIP at 4q31, IREB2 and nicotinic acetylcholine receptors (CHRNA3 and CHRNA5) o at 15q25, the 19q13 locus with RAB4B, EGLN2, and CYP2A6, RIN3 at 14q32, MMP12 at 11q22, and TGFB2 at 1q41 [5–8]. Epigenetic changes includes, but are not limited to, posttranslational modifications of histones, DNA methylation, and RNA modification, which regulate gene expression without altering the gene sequence. Screening of miRNA and mRNA profiles in lung samples from smokers with or without COPD revealed that 70 miRNAs and 2667 mRNA differentially expressed. Several miRNAs, including members of the miR15/107 family, were found to regulate TGF-β signaling in COPD [9]. DNA methylation is an important regulator of gene expression, which is strongly regulated by environmental factors. DNA methylation analysis of small airway epithelia from COPD subjects found 1120 differentially methylated genes, mostly hypermethylated, which showed enrichment for three pathways: G-protein-coupled receptor signaling, arene receptor signaling, and cAMP-mediated signaling. The methylation status of 144 genes was negatively correlated with gene expression, which involved in phosphatase and tensin homolog (PTEN) signaling, the nuclear factor erythroid-derived 2-related factor 2 (also known as Nrf2) oxidative stress response, and the effect of IL-17F on allergic inflammatory diseases [10]. The emerging role of epigenetics in the development of COPD will make it possible to reprogram, minimize risk, explain causes, and create new treatments for COPD.

3. Diagnosis of COPD

Patients with dyspnea, chronic cough and/or expectoration, a history of recurrent lower respiratory tract infections, and/or a history of exposure to risk factors are considered as COPD. Pulmonary function tests are necessary to confirm the diagnosis of COPD, such as forced expiratory volume in 1 second/forced vital capacity, FEV1/FVC < 0.70 after inhalation of bronchodilator, which can confirm the presence of persistent airflow limitation. Lung function assessed by forced expiratory volume in 1 second (FEV1), forced vital capacity (FVC), and the ratio of FEV1 to FVC (FEV1/FVC) reflect the physiological state of the lung, and these indices can be used to diagnose and monitor COPD. The goal of COPD assessment is to determine the degree of airflow limitation, the impact of the disease on the patient's health, and the risk of long-term adverse outcomes (such as AECOPD, hospitalization, or death) to guide treatment. Spirometer is an important examination instrument for the diagnosis of COPD. Clinically, it is necessary to find indicators that can predict the occurrence and development of airflow limitation and comprehensively evaluate the respiratory physiology of COPD. Alveolar diffusion is the process of gas molecules exchange through the alveolar membrane (alveolar-capillary membrane). DLco was measured by single breath method to reflect the pulmonary diffusion function. Respiratory physiological indicators other than portable pulmonary function instruments can be supplemented to better assess COPD.

Recent studies have suggested that COPD may be caused by a decreased peak and/or an accelerated decline in lung function in early adulthood. COPD can start early in life and take a long time to manifest itself clinically, so identifying "early" COPD is difficult. In addition, the biological "early" associated with the initial mechanisms that ultimately lead to COPD should be distinguished from the clinical "early," which reflects the initial perception of symptoms, functional limitations, and/or noted structural abnormalities. Pulmonary function tests are poorly correlated with clinical characteristics and lack sufficient sensitivity for early diagnosis. Meanwhile, due to the heterogeneity and phenotypic complexity of COPD, pulmonary function measurements provide limited information on prognosis, predictive outcome, and treatment strategy, which are not sufficient for accurate diagnosis, treatment, and efficacy evaluation. Patients with COPD often suffer from cardiovascular disease, skeletal muscle dysfunction, metabolic syndrome, osteoporosis, depression, anxiety, lung cancer, and other diseases. In view of the fact that these complications are independent risk factors for hospitalization and death, we should actively look for complications and give correct treatment to patients with COPD. The development of high-throughput technologies such as genomics, proteomics, and metabolomics has provided effective tools for elucidating global changes in complex inflammatory diseases such as COPD. Among them, COPD "omics" research mainly focuses on DNA (genetic) and RNA (transcriptome) markers. The advent of mass spectrometry (MS), including gas chromatography/MS and liquid chromatography/MS, has made proteomics and metabolomics more feasible for large-scale population studies. The multi-omics integration study by similarity network fusion significantly improved the accuracy of grouping COPD patients from healthy nonsmokers to smokers with normal lung capacity, indicating that multi-omics integration data can improve the accuracy of COPD diagnosis and help promote the understanding of its pathogenesis.

3.1 Metabonomics

Metabonomics is a comprehensive assessment of low-molecular-weight (< 1000 Da) endogenous metabolites, which can reflect biochemical reactions and metabolic changes under given physiological or pathophysiological conditions. Endogenous metabolites include a variety of small molecules such as sugars, lipids, steroids, and amino acids. The expression of these metabolites in humans represents the functional phenotype of cell, organ, or tissue. Metabonomics is of great help in identifying disease-related metabolites. Through the detection of various biological fluids (blood, urine, bronchoalveolar lavage fluid), it can provide help for the early detection of complex diseases and in-depth understanding of the pathogenesis of diseases. Smoking increases levels of nicotine and its metabolites, but also has a strong effect on the systemic metabolism of amino acids, lipids, and other small molecules. A study that recruited 211 subjects with COPD found that peripheral blood monocyte sphingolipid pathway enzyme expression and plasma small molecules such as ceramide were biomarkers of COPD and emphysema, even after adjustment for smoking. Subsequent targeted plasma metabolomics studies in 129 subjects with COPD genes further identified five sphingomyelins associated with emphysema and four trihexosylceramides and three dihexosylceramides associated with COPD exacerbations [11]. These findings support sphingolipids as potential new therapeutic targets for emphysema. Urine is also a common and available sample for metabolomics studies. Urine metabolomics is less invasive to participants than serum/plasma because serum metabolites remain relatively constant due to the balance of metabolism in the body, and urine samples are more suitable for metabolomics differential analysis than blood. Urine profiles of COPD patients and healthy controls were successfully isolated with ultrahigh performance liquid chromatography/MS (UPLC/MS)-based metabolomics. Ten metabolic biomarkers associated with COPD were identified in urine samples involving amino acid metabolism, lipid and fatty acid metabolism, and glucose metabolism. Amino acid metabolism is related to nutritional status, oxidative stress, and inflammatory response. Muscle dysfunction is an important feature of COPD patients, particularly during cachexia. In COPD patients, the concentration of histidine is increased, and muscle is synthesized by methyltransferase conversion to methylhistidine during cross-linking of actin and inosine [12]. Reduced use of histidine for muscle growth may result in increased serum histidine levels. In COPD patients, branched-chain amino acids (BCAAs) have been reduced; BCAAs regulate protein production and glucose homeostasis by continuously delivering BCAAs to skeletal muscle [13]. The reduction of BCAAs in COPD may indicate the risk of protein malnutrition. For underweight COPD patients, hypermetabolism caused by COPD exacerbation and respiratory muscle weakness is the main reason for the decline of BCAA concentration. However, the hydrolysis of muscle proteins and the consumption of branched-chain amino acids are part of the basic physiological function of providing carbon for gluconeogenesis during fasting. Cachexia patients with weight loss show increased gluconeogenesis [14], which will lead to increased consumption and decreased content of BCAAs in humans.

3.2 Proteomics

Proteomics aims to identify potential protein biomarkers of disease and has become a popular tool for both basic and clinical research. Proteomics has the potential to reveal some disease mechanisms that cannot be determined at the genomic level and has the great advantage of direct clinical relevance. Proteomic approaches have been used in many chronic lung diseases, such as cystic fibrosis, idiopathic pulmonary fibrosis (IPF), sarcoidosis, asthma, and so on. With the development of analysis and detection technology, the identification of potential protein biomarkers can be achieved in COPD research. Plasma proteins are involved in inflammation, coagulation regulation, lipid metabolism, and oxidative stress, and changes between healthy people and mild COPD can be evaluated at an early stage of the disease, helping us to identify early COPD. Currently, the most promising blood biomarker for COPD is sRAGE. sRAGE is an isoform of the advanced glycation end product (RAGE) transmembrane receptor that lacks a transmembrane domain through proteolytic cleavage. RAGE is encoded by the AGER gene, and SNPs in AGER have been associated with COPD and emphysema in targeted and genome-wide association studies [15]. RAGE binds damage-associated molecular pattern molecules to perpetuate inflammation in lung epithelial cells. In COPDGene, subjects with more severe emphysema had lower plasma sRAGE. The SNP in AGER (rs2070600) was associated with lower sRAGE plasma levels in COPDGene and other cohorts. Plasma sRAGE is a predictor of emphysema progressions, and it will be the first blood biomarker for emphysema to be submitted to the US Food and Drug Administration and the European Medicines Agency Biomarker Certification Program [16, 17]. While sRAGE is currently the best biomarker for emphysema, blood markers of inflammation are also associated with COPD severity and progression. In a study of 2123 subjects from COPDgene and 1117 subjects from SPIROMICS, plasma IL-6 and IL-8 were found to be positively associated with emphysema progression, but not with COPD severity and smoking status [18]. The detection of proteins in BALF and EBC can also help to clarify the pathogenesis of COPD and lung defense mechanism. In order to obtain an accurate diagnosis of COPD, an invasive approach is required in some cases. Lung tissue sample obtained by transbronchial lung biopsy or open lung biopsy procedure can also be used to analyze proteomic changes. Comparisons of lung tissues from COPD patients and healthy controls using MALDI-TOF-MS revealed significantly higher levels of matrix ferroproteinase-13 (MMP-13) and thioredoxin-like 2 in COPD patients, which may be more closely associated with the development of airflow limitation. In COPD patients, the level of SP-a in lung tissue was increased, and the level of SP-a in induced sputum supernatant was increased, but the levels of other surfactant proteins (SP-B, SPC, SP-D) were not changed. These results suggest that SP-a may be involved in the pathogenesis of COPD. However, the determination of a protein as a biomarker requires a large amount of sample data as a basis. We still have a lot of work to do.

3.3 Transcriptomics

The aim of transcriptome analysis is to capture coding and non-coding RNAs and quantify the heterogeneity of gene expression in cells, tissues, organs, and even the whole body. Transcriptomics can provide functional characterization and annotation of genes/genomes previously revealed by DNA sequencing [19]. Currently, three transcriptomics-related technologies are employed, including real-time quantitative PCR (qPCR), microarray, and RNA sequencing. The sample sources for the COPD transcriptomics study were focused on peripheral blood, lung tissue, and sputum. Similar to the epigenome, the transcriptome can be influenced by factors such as age, gender, cell type, environmental exposure, and disease status. For example, a study conducted microarray gene expression profiling of peripheral blood mononuclear cells collected from 136 COPDGene subjects and found that 1090 transcripts associated with FEV 1% prediction and 1745 transcripts associated with FEV 1/FVC, genes that overrepresent pathways associated with immunity, inflammatory response, and sphingolipid (ceramide) metabolism and signaling. At single cell level, COPD was found to be associated with a decreased ratio of specific transcriptome features of CD4+ resting memory cells and naive B cells [20]. There are also studies using gene expression profiling of lung tissue to explore the molecular pathogenesis of early COPD with emphysema. RNASeq was used to detect 16,676 genes expressed in lung tissue. Among them, 1226 genes in the COPD group with emphysema and 434 genes in the non-emphysema group were differentially expressed with healthy smokers [21]. Xiao et al. explored the relationship between gene transcriptomics and several single-nucleotide polymorphisms in sputum. Distal gene loci and biomarker encoding genes may influence circulating levels of COPD-associated pneumonia proteins, and a subset of these protein quantitative trait loci may influence their susceptibility in the lung and/or COPD. A notable feature of transcriptomics research is that the number of potential transcription variables is usually very large, and special methods are needed to deal with the huge and disordered data. For example, the weighted gene co-expression network and clustering method can be used to reduce the dimensionality.

COPD exacerbations are highly heterogeneous events associated with increased airway and systemic inflammation and physiologic changes, and reliable and objective biomarkers are invaluable to aid diagnosis and guide appropriate treatment. In blood, urine, breath samples (including exhaled breath, sputum, bronchoalveolar lavage fluid, and bronchial biopsies), levels of various immune inflammatory cells and molecules are elevated, such as CRP, PCT, BNP, plasma fibrinogen, IL-6, sputum eosinophilia, IL1β, CXCL10 (IP-10), some of which have been used in clinical examinations to assist in the evaluation of COPD deterioration [22]. At present, the research on the pathogenesis of AECOPD is still insufficient, and there are contradictory conclusions. In recent years, the widespread use of high-throughput sequencing technology has enabled us to study COPD in greater depth. At the metabolomics level, newly discovered markers of differential metabolism may be associated with disease states; at the proteomics level, several disease-related proteins have been identified and are expected to be used in the early diagnosis of COPD, while in transcriptomics, some biomarkers may be used to evaluate the prognosis of the disease. In general, multi-omics studies provide a way to discover biomarkers for early diagnosis of COPD, but the identified prospective biomarkers need to be clinically validated for early diagnosis of COPD. Therefore, clinicians need to collect a large number of patient data and clinical samples. Only by combining proteomics, transcriptomics, metabolomics, and bioinformatics, can we obtain reliable and helpful results for clinical diagnosis and treatment.

4. Research progress on prevention and management of COPD

4.1 Smoking cessation

Smoking cessation is the first step in the treatment of COPD and the key to reducing the progressive decline of lung function. Lung function and smoking-related comorbidities (lung cancer and cardiovascular disease) increase mortality rate over time in COPD patients. Cooking with stoves instead of open fires can reduce the progressive decline in lung function by reducing indoor air pollution in a manner similar to smoking cessation. It is different for COPD patients with high tobacco dependence to smoking cessation. Thus, up to 40% of patients, even those with severe COPD, are persistent smokers. Drug therapy and nicotine replacement therapy can improve long-term abstinence rates. Smoking legislation and counseling by medical professionals can also improve abstinence rates. Currently, the effectiveness and safety of e-cigarettes as a smoking cessation aid are uncertain.

4.2 Physical activity

Increasing physical activity of daily living is as important as smoking cessation in reducing morbidity and mortality rate in COPD patients. In the early stage of the disease, lack of physical activity is closely related to hospitalization and mortality. In COPD patients, walking for 15 minutes per day reduced the risk of death by 14%, and an increase of 600 steps per day was associated with a lower risk of hospitalization. GOLD 2022 introduces the meta-analysis that included a total of 23 studies with 1663 participants. Compared with other groups, the mean deviation of 6 minutes walking distance (6MWD), FEV1 as a percentage of predicted values, SGRQ scores, and Chronic Respiratory Disease Questionnaire (CRQ) scores in Tai Chi group were significantly improved [23]. Tai Chi may have the potential to reduce dyspnea, improve exercise ability and quality of life in patients with COPD. Patients with COPD may benefit from practicing Tai Chi, but more effective programs need to be further studied.

4.3 Pulmonary rehabilitation

"Rehabilitation 2030" is a new strategic approach to prioritizing and strengthening rehabilitation services in the health system. As part of the WHO initiative, a series of rehabilitation interventions is being developed that includes pulmonary rehabilitation for COPD. Inpatient or outpatient pulmonary rehabilitation for patients with COPD is effective in improving multiple clinically relevant outcomes. There is evidence that the core components of pulmonary rehabilitation, including exercise training combined with disease-specific education and self-management interventions, can benefit almost every COPD patient.

Pulmonary rehabilitation is an effective multidisciplinary treatment strategy that improves dyspnea, exercise tolerance, and health-related quality of life. Classical exercise programs with individualized endurance and strength training remain the cornerstone of pulmonary rehabilitation, and education to promote behavior change and self-management are also necessary for successful intervention. Tele-rehabilitation has been proposed as an alternative to traditional methods. The results of multiple trials conducted in groups and individuals with multiple tele-rehabilitation delivery platforms (videoconferencing, telephone-only, websites with telephone support, mobile applications with feedback, centralized "hubs" for people to gather) show that tele-rehabilitation is safe and has similar benefits to center-based respiratory rehabilitation in a range of outcomes [24]. However, the evidence is still evolving and best practices have not yet been established.

4.4 Pharmacotherapy

Medical therapy for COPD is used to reduce symptoms, decrease the frequency and severity of exacerbations, and improve exercise tolerance and health. Maintenance drug therapy in the stable phase aims to improve symptoms, improve health-related quality of life, improve exercise intolerance, and reduce the risk of deterioration. In terms of airflow restriction, reduction of air entrapment, and improvement of exercise intolerance, inhaled long-acting beta2 agonists (LABAs) and long-acting muscarinic antagonists (LAMAs) have similar effects. LAMA tiotropium appears to be superior to LABA in preventing exacerbations and is as effective as the combination of inhaled corticosteroids and LABA. Therefore, LAMA monotherapy should be superior to LABA monotherapy in patients with a history of exacerbation. Acute exacerbations occurred significantly less during LABA-LAMA (indacaterol-glycopyrrolate) therapy than during LAMA (glycopyrrolate) monotherapy. Besides, the addition of LAMA and inhaled corticosteroids to LABA resulted in less aggravation than LABA and inhaled corticosteroids alone. Clinicians are concerned about whether further escalation from LABA-LAMA to triple therapy consisting of LABA, LAMA, and inhaled corticosteroids will provide additional benefits. Two large-scale studies found that triple therapy (LABA/LAMA/ICS) can reduce the death rate of COPD [25, 26]. For the benefit of fixed triple therapy for AECOPD, ETHOS research published evidence-based medicine evidence in the New England Journal of Medicine in June 2020. In this study, 8578 patients with chronic COPD were enrolled, aged 40 ~ 80 years, with smoking history of ≥10 packs/year, cat score ≥ 10 points, maintenance treatment with ≥2 inhalants before screening, maintenance treatment time ≥ 6 weeks, FEV1 estimated value ≥25% and < 65%, and moderate or severe AECOPD history 12 months before screening; To compare the efficacy and safety of budesonide/glulomonium bromide/formforminhaled aerosol (MDI) and dual therapy (bud/form and gly/form) with two ICs doses, all cause death was the secondary endpoint; compared with laba/lama, the use of triple therapy containing high-dose ICs (not low-dose ICs) is associated with lower mortality. The results of this study have important clinical significance, and further research or analysis may help to determine whether specific patient subgroups show greater survival benefits. The potential benefit of reducing acute exacerbation by adding inhaled corticosteroids to LABA needs to be judged and weighed the potential risk of pneumonia. When fluticasone, an inhaled corticosteroid, is added to LABA, COPD patients with low eosinophil counts may have an increased risk of pneumonia. This suggests that there is a subgroup with a high eosinophil count, and the benefits of inhaled corticosteroids outweigh the risks. Clinicians must judge whether glucocorticoid treatment needs to be combined or stopped according to the clinical symptoms, acute exacerbation risk, asthma, bronchiectasis, pulmonary tuberculosis, blood eosinophils, and other indicators of patients, and select the route, dose, and course of glucocorticoid administration according to the heterogeneity of AECOPD. Eosinophils can predict the risk of acute exacerbation, and ICS has guiding value in preventing future AECOPD. The survey data showed that the blood eosinophil count was <100 cells/μl of COPD patients who were less likely to benefit from the treatment with the treatment plan containing ICS. In addition, the presence of Proteus, Haemophilus, and increased bacterial infections and pneumonia was associated with lower blood and sputum eosinophil counts. Therefore, a lower blood eosinophil count can identify characteristic individuals of the microbiome with an increased risk of clinical deterioration caused by pathogenic bacteria. Higher blood eosinophils and lung eosinophils in COPD patients were associated with higher levels of type 2 airway inflammation markers. These differences in airway inflammation may explain the different responses of eosinophils to ICS therapy. The estimated value of eosinophil whose number is <100cells/μl and ≥ 300 cells/μl can be used to predict the different probability of treatment benefit. It should be noted that the use of eosinophils, which can predict the efficacy of ICS, should always be combined with clinical assessment of the risk of acute exacerbation. In the population with low ICS use rate, a greater decrease in FEV1 was observed in mild to moderate COPD patients with high blood eosinophil count, which indicates that blood eosinophils can be used as a biomarker of decreased lung function and are not affected by ICS use. In young persons without COPD, higher eosinophil counts were associated with an increased risk of subsequent COPD [27]. In conclusion, blood eosinophils can help clinicians evaluate the possibility of beneficial preventive response to the addition of ICS to conventional bronchodilator therapy. Therefore, blood eosinophils count can be used as biomarkers combined with clinical evaluation when making decisions about the use of ICS. In view of the increasing importance of clinical features and individualized treatment decisions, further treatment options for this subgroup should be carefully examined. Bronchodilator therapy (LABA, LAMA, or a combination of both) has been proved to be generally safe in randomized controlled trials. However, owing to these trials usually excluding patients who have severe heart disease, clinicians should be aware of the cardiac events reported in meta-analysis and observational studies. Patients reported that symptoms of chronic bronchitis may benefit from the addition of oral phosphodiesterase 4 inhibitor roflukast, especially those who have been hospitalized for COPD deterioration or have received more than two deterioration treatments in the outpatient department. Macrolide therapy is recommended for long-term and low-dose use in patients who have smoked. However, it is necessary to consider the side effects associated with propenolactone, the uncertainty of treatment for more than 1 year, and the resistance of bacteria to macrolides. The World Health Organization (WHO) has formulated the necessary intervention measures for COPD in low- and middle-income countries, and it pointed out that if the symptoms persist, low-dose theophylline can be added according to drug availability. Gold2022 suggests that FEV1 accounts for 35% ~ 60% of the estimated value, and COPD patients with smoking history are the best subjects for α 1 antitrypsin deficiency (AATD) augmentation therapy (evidence level B). The existing clinical trials and registration data are almost completely concentrated on patients with ZZ (ZZAATD/PiZZ) genotype. Recent studies have shown that the risk of mild COPD in Z gene heterozygotes is increased. Different from ZZ genotype, Z gene heterozygotes will not develop COPD in the condition of non-smoking. Therefore, it is considered that quitting smoking can prevent the development of this kind of patients [28].

There are limitations in the evidence base of drug therapy for COPD. Almost all drug treatment studies included patients who had smoked for at least 10 years and excluded patients with asthma. It is not clear how effective COPD drugs are in patients who have never smoked or who have asthma. Due to the complexity of airway inflammation and related clinical phenotypes in COPD, a single inflammatory pathway or mechanism may not be enough to continuously inhibit inflammation in all patients with COPD. Each drug treatment plan should be individualized according to the severity of COPD symptoms, the risk of acute exacerbation, adverse reactions, complications, the availability and cost of drugs, as well as the patient's response, preference, and ability to use various drug delivery devices.

4.5 Interventional treatments

For some patients with advanced emphysema whose medical treatment is ineffective, surgery or bronchoscopic intervention may benefit. Individualized treatment decisions should be based on the characteristics of emphysema, such as heterogeneous and homogeneous, complete lobar fissure or collateral ventilation. For most patients, the therapeutic effect needs to be combined with potential complications such as pneumothorax and pneumonia. Other interventions, including hot steam or sclerotherapy, can show some efficacy, but may lead to more complications. For patients with advanced COPD, lung transplantation is still an option to improve the quality of life and exercise endurance, but it has no effect on the overall survival rate. Palliative treatment is an effective method to control the late COPD symptoms.

4.6 Oxygen and ventilatory support

For patients with stable COPD and moderate decline of oxygenation index when they rest or exercise, long-term oxygen therapy should not be conducted routinely, but individual factors of patients must be considered when evaluating patients' demand for supplemental oxygen. For patients with severe resting hypoxemia ([pao2] $\leq$ 55 mmHg) or moderate hypoxemia (PaO2 $\leq$ 60 mmHg) and signs of heart failure, pulmonary hypertension, or polycythemia, long-term oxygen therapy can improve their survival rate. The application of transnasal high flow oxygen therapy (HFNC) in the rehabilitation of COPD is a hot spot in recent years. A meta-analysis from 10 RCTs compared HFNC with conventional oxygen therapy (COT) or NIV in improving respiratory rate, FEV1, tidal volume, oxygen partial pressure, total SGRQ score, 6MWD, and exercise tolerance time [29]. The comprehensive data of six studies showed that the respiratory rate of COPD patients in HFNC group was lower. The comprehensive data of three studies showed that FEV1 of HFNC group was lower. There was no difference in tidal volume between patients with COPD in HFNC group and control group; There was no significant improvement in oxygen partial pressure between HFNC group and control group. In the subgroup analysis of HFNC and COT, the total score of SGRQ in HFNC group increased. Two multicenter RCTs showed an increase in 6MWD after HFNC, but no increase in exercise tolerance time. The differences in evidence quality included in this meta-analysis are prominent, which indicate that more high-quality RCTs are needed to verify these evidences. For patients with stable hypercapnia and high inspiratory pressure, noninvasive positive pressure ventilation aims to reduce the partial pressure of carbon dioxide ($PaCO_2$) in arterial blood by at least 20% or lower than 6.5 kPa, which can improve the survival rate. Therefore, patients who meet the condition and have a special home care environment can consider this method.

4.7 Treatment of comorbidities

Comorbidities affect a large part of patients with COPD. A cluster analysis was conducted on 213 COPD patients, and five unique clusters of comorbidities were established: (1) fewer comorbidities; (2) cardiovascular clusters, including hypertension and atherosclerosis, (3) cachexia clusters, including low body mass index (BMI), muscle atrophy, osteoporosis, and impairment of renal function; (4) metabolic clusters, including high BMI, dyslipidemia, hypertension, and atherosclerosis sclerosis; (5) psychological cluster, including anxiety and depression. Cardiovascular disease is a common and important complication of COPD. Although the lung function is similar, there are important differences in dyspnea and quality of life in different clusters. Systemic inflammation in cardiovascular and metabolic clusters is at a high level. Lung cancer is common in COPD patients and is the leading cause of death. The United States Preventive Services Task Force (USPSTF) updated its recommendations for lung cancer screening in 2021,which recommend that conduct LDCT annual lung cancer screening for adults aged 50 ~ 80 who have 20 packs per year of smoking history and currently smoke or quit smoking within the past 15 years [30]. Osteoporosis and depression/anxiety are common complications of COPD, which are often missed, and are related to poor health status and prognosis. Gastroesophageal reflux is associated with increased risk of AECOPD and poor health. Overall, COPD combined with other that has a great impact on the prognosis. The existence of comorbidities should not change the treatment plan of COPD, and the comorbidities should be treated according to the conventional standard, which has nothing to do with the existence of COPD. When COPD is part of a multi-disease care plan, attention should be paid to ensuring the simplicity of treatment and minimizing multidrug treatment. Some drugs for COPD have been evaluated as well as the effects of treatment outside the lung. The inhaled combination of fluticasone furoate and viranterol (an inhaled corticosteroid and a LABA) did not affect mortality or cardiovascular outcomes in patients with moderate COPD and increased risk of cardiovascular disease, but it improved cardiac insufficiency associated with hyperinflation. In a meta-analysis, there were fewer major cardiovascular events after roflukast treatment, but no randomized controlled study has been conducted to test the potential benefits of roflukast treatment on cardiovascular outcomes in COPD.

4.8 Treatment of exacerbations of COPD

Exacerbation of COPD is an acute exacerbation of respiratory symptoms (dyspnea, cough, expectoration, and suppuration) that requires a change in treatment strategy. AECOPD can be caused by a variety of factorshe, and the most common cause is viral or bacterial respiratory tract infection. Patients are often hospitalized with dyspnea as the main symptom. The exacerbation of respiratory symptoms in COPD patients needs to be identified as AECOPD or other causes. One important differential diagnosis is pulmonary embolism (PE). In a study that included 740 AECOPD patients, 44 patients were diagnosed with PE within 48 hours after being admitted to hospital [31]. Among the 670 patients who were considered to have no venous thromboembolism and did not receive anticoagulant therapy at the time of admission, five patients developed PE during the follow-up period, of which three patients developed PE related death. The overall case fatality rate in 3 months was 6.8%. In the patients with COPD admitted due to acute deterioration of respiratory symptoms, 5.9% detected PE using predefined diagnostic algorithms. Further studies are needed to understand the possible role of systematic screening for PE in this patient population. At the same time, cardiovascular events and pneumonia also need to be excluded during acute attack. The deterioration negatively affects lung function decline, health-related quality of life, and prognosis. The treatment goal of ECOPD is to minimize the adverse effects caused by this acute exacerbation and prevent the occurrence of acute exacerbation in the future. Recommended single-use short effect β receptor agonists with or without short acting anticholinergic drugs are the initial treatment for AECOPD. Short-term systemic glucocorticoid therapy (e.g., 40 mg prednisone for 5 days) with or without short course antibiotics is the preferred treatment for acute episode events. Severe exacerbations require hospitalization and individualized treatment, including noninvasive ventilation support (preferred), oxygen therapy, treatment of associated diseases (such as heart failure, pneumonia), and finally, weaning or invasive ventilation. Cohort studies have shown that more than half of AECOPD patients have cardiovascular disease. Even without clinical symptoms of cardiac involvement, biochemical evidence of cardiac dysfunction (such as high concentration of troponin I or B-type natriuretic peptide) is common during treatment. About 20% of AECOPD may be due to the deterioration of underlying cardiovascular disease, and such patients have poor prognosis after admission. In Europe, 11% of patients died within 90 days after admission. The hospital stay of 50% of the patients was extended to 3 months; 35% of the patients were readmitted within 90 days. Gold2022 gives discharge criteria and follow-up recommendations: record the ability to perform physical activities during the follow-up of 1–4 weeks and consider whether the patient is suitable for participating in lung rehabilitation, at the same time, increasing protective measures such as wearing masks, reducing social contact, and washing hands frequently can reduce the frequency of AECOPD.

4.9 Vaccination

It is generally recommended that COPD patients receive influenza vaccine and pneumococcal vaccine. Influenza vaccine can reduce the incidence of lower respiratory tract infection; S. pneumoniae vaccine can reduce lower respiratory tract infection and prevent acute exacerbation of COPD. The Centers for Disease Control and prevention of the United States recommended supplementary vaccination for the patients with COPD who are not vaccinated with Tdap vaccine (dtap/dtpa) to prevent the occurrence of pertussis, tetanus, and diphtheria, in addition recommended that patients aged 50 and over with COPD should be vaccinated with herpes zoster vaccine. Novel coronavirus vaccine can effectively prevent SARS-CoV-2 infection. Patients with COPD should be vaccinated with novel coronavirus vaccine according to the national recommendations.

4.10 Brief summary

Due to the complex and heterogeneous COPD, there are individual differences in its clinical management. To this end, scientists have proposed a management strategy based on treatable characteristics (TTs), which can identify TTs according to their clinical characteristics (phenotype) and/or through effective biomarkers of specific pathological mechanisms (endotype) in the lung, extrapulmonary, and behavioral/environmental domains. TTs can coexist, interact, and change over time in the same patient (either spontaneously or as a result of treatment). Because TTs-guided management can improve clinical outcomes, the design of future trials for the treatment of early-onset patients needs to consider the presence or absence of TTs. Again, it is important to note that since endomorphs may differ with age, it may be different in early-onset and elderly patients, and the better understanding gained from the current study of early-onset COPD patients may provide guidance for future treatment guidelines.

5. Conclusion

Chronic obstructive pulmonary disease (COPD), as a common and heterogeneous respiratory disease, is characterized by persistent and incomplete reversible airflow limitation. Due to the heterogeneity and phenotypic complexity of COPD, traditional diagnostic methods can only provide limited predictive outcome and treatment information, which is insufficient for accurate diagnosis and evaluation. With the development of omics technology in recent years, genomics, proteomics, and metabolomics are widely used in the study of COPD, providing good tools for the discovery of biomarkers for diagnosis and elucidation of the complex mechanisms of COPD. In this chapter, based on the risk factors and causes of COPD, combined with metabolomics, proteomics, and transcriptomics studies reported in recent years, possible biomarkers for the diagnosis of COPD are summarized. It is expected to explore important metabolites and proteins involved in important pathways of COPD progression through protein-protein interaction and multi-omics analysis to explain the pathogenesis of COPD. Finally, the prospects and challenges of COPD diagnosis and treatment research are put forward. In the foreseeable future, on a global scale, COPD will remain a major public health problem. Population development in high-income countries and a significant increase in NCDs in low-income countries will accelerate this health burden, with risk factors largely unchanged. A better understanding of the genetic molecules and biology of the different endomorphs and phenotypes of this disease is needed to enable the development of innovative drugs.

Funding

This work was supported by the National Natural Science Foundation of China (81970026, 82000029), Chengdu High-level Key Clinical Specialty Construction Project (ZX20201202020), Chengdu Science and Technology Bureau (2021-YF09–00102-SN).

Author details

Lei Zhang[1,2†], Xiang He[1,2†*], Jiliu Liu[1,2], Yi Zhang[1,2], Xiaohui Zuo[1,2] and Guoping Li[1,2*]

1 Laboratory of Allergy and Precision Medicine, Chengdu Institute of Respiratory Health, The Third People's Hospital of Chengdu, Affiliated Hospital of Southwest Jiaotong University, Chengdu, China

2 Department of Pulmonary and Critical Care Medicine, Chengdu Third People's Hospital Branch of National Clinical Research Center for Respiratory Disease, Affiliated Hospital of ChongQing Medical University, Chengdu, China

*Address all correspondence to: xiangge530@hotmail.com; lzlgp@163.com

† These authors contributed equally to this work.

References

[1] Hammond EE et al. The global impact of aspergillus infection on COPD. BMC Pulmonary Medicine. 2020;**20**(1):241

[2] Tabyshova A et al. Gaps in COPD guidelines of low- and middle-income countries: A systematic scoping review. Chest. 2021;**159**(2):575-584

[3] Huang YJ et al. Airway microbiome dynamics in exacerbations of chronic obstructive pulmonary disease. Journal of Clinical Microbiology. 2014;**52**(8):2813-2823

[4] Eltboli O et al. COPD exacerbation severity and frequency is associated with impaired macrophage efferocytosis of eosinophils. BMC Pulmonary Medicine. 2014;**14**(1):1-10

[5] Hobbs BD, Hersh CP. Integrative genomics of chronic obstructive pulmonary disease. Biochemical & Biophysical Research Communications. 2014;**452**(2):276-286

[6] Pan et al. Relationships of COX2 and MMP12 genetic polymorphisms with chronic obstructive pulmonary disease risk: A meta-analysis. Molecular Biology Reports. 2015;**42**(10):1491-1491

[7] Xie ZK et al. Association between the IL1B, IL1RN polymorphisms and COPD risk: A meta-analysis. Scientific Reports. 2014;**4**:6202

[8] Liang S et al. A disintegrin and metalloprotease 33 (ADAM33) gene polymorphisms and the risk of asthma: A meta-analysis. Human Immunology. 2013;**74**(5):648-657

[9] Ezzie ME et al. Gene expression networks in COPD: microRNA and mRNA regulation. Thorax. 2012;**67**(2):122-131

[10] Vucic EA et al. DNA methylation is globally disrupted and associated with expression changes in chronic obstructive pulmonary disease small airways. American Journal of Respiratory Cell and Molecular Biology. 2014;**50**(5):912-922

[11] Bowler RP et al. Plasma sphingolipids associated with chronic obstructive pulmonary disease phenotypes. American Journal of Respiratory & Critical Care Medicine. 2015;**191**(3):275-284

[12] Wang CH et al. Amino acid-based metabolic panel provides robust prognostic value additive to b-natriuretic peptide and traditional risk factors in heart failure. Disease Markers. 2018;**2018**:3784589

[13] Fontana L et al. Decreased consumption of branched-chain amino acids improves metabolic health. Cell Reports.2016;**16**(2):520-530

[14] Yoneda T et al. Plasma levels of amino acids and hypermetabolism in patients with chronic obstructive pulmonary disease. Nutrition. 2001;**17**(2):95-99

[15] Cheng DT et al. Systemic soluble receptor for advanced glycation endproducts is a biomarker of emphysema and associated with AGER genetic variants in patients with chronic obstructive pulmonary disease. American Journal of Respiratory and Critical Care Medicine. 2013;**188**(8):948-957

[16] Hurst JR et al. Evaluation of COPD longitudinally to identify predictive surrogate endpoints (ECLIPSE) investigators. Susceptibility to exacerbation in chronic obstructive pulmonary disease. The New England Journal of Medicine. 2010;**363**(12):1128-1138

[17] Coxson HO et al. The presence and progression of emphysema in COPD as determined by CT scanning and biomarker expression: A prospective analysis from the ECLIPSE study. Lancet Respiratory Medicine. 2013;**1**(2):129-136

[18] Eric et al. The value of blood cytokines and chemokines in assessing COPD. Respiratory Research. 2017;**18**(1):180

[19] Shendure J, Ji H. Next-generation DNA sequencing. Nature Biotechnology. 2008;**26**(10):1135-1145

[20] Halper-Stromberg et al. Systemic markers of adaptive and innate immunity are associated with chronic obstructive pulmonary disease severity and Spirometric disease progression. American Journal of Respiratory Cell and Molecular Biology. 2018;**58**(4):500-509

[21] Ina J et al. Gene expression profile of human lung in a relatively early stage of COPD with emphysema. International Journal of COPD. 2018;**13**:2643-2655

[22] Saito J et al. Sputum-to-serum hydrogen sulfide ratio in COPD. Thorax. 2014;**69**(10):903-909

[23] Liu X et al. The effect of tai chi on the pulmonary rehabilitation of chronic obstructive pulmonary disease: A systematic review and meta-analysis. Annals of Palliative Medicine. 2021;**10**(4):3763-3782

[24] Cox NS et al. Telerehabilitation for chronic respiratory disease. Cochrane Database of Systematic Reviews. 2021;**1**(1):CD013040

[25] Martinez FJ et al. Benefits of budesonide/glycopyrrolate/ formoterol fumarate (BGF) on symptoms and quality of life in patients with COPD in the ETHOS trial. Respiratory Medicine. 2021;**185**:106509

[26] Lipson DA et al. Reduction in all-cause mortality with fluticasone Furoate/Umeclidinium/Vilanterol in COPD patients. American Journal of Respiratory and Critical Care Medicine. 2020;**201**(12):1508-1516

[27] Park HY, Chang Y, Kang D, Hong YS, Zhao D, Ahn J, et al. Blood eosinophil counts and the development of obstructive lung disease: The Kangbuk Samsung Health Study. European Respiratory Journal. 2021;**58**(4):2003823

[28] Franciosi AN et al. Clarifying the risk of lung disease in SZ α1-antitrypsin deficiency. American Journal of Respiratory and Critical Care Medicine. 2020;**202**(1):73-82

[29] Fu C et al. Efficiency of high-flow nasal cannula on pulmonary rehabilitation in COPD patients: A meta-analysis. BioMed Research International. 2020;**2020**(2016):1-9

[30] Potter AL et al. The 2021 USPSTF lung cancer screening guidelines: A new frontier. Lancet Respiratory Medicine. Jul 2021;**9**(7):689-691

[31] Couturaud F et al. Prevalence of pulmonary embolism among patients with COPD hospitalized with acutely worsening respiratory symptoms. JAMA The Journal of the American Medical Association. 2021;**325**(1):59

Chapter 3

COPD and Inflammation

Christian Peiser

Abstract

COPD is associated with chronic inflammation of the airways, which causes damage to defense and repair mechanisms, resulting in remodeling processes in the bronchi and bronchioles. This leads to fibrosis of the lung tissue, increased smooth muscle tension, swelling of bronchial mucosa, loss of cilia function with accumulation of mucus, and finally to chronic pulmonary obstruction and possibly emphysema, with the main symptoms of dyspnea, coughing, and expectoration. Inhaled pollutants can activate immune cells like macrophages, T-lymphocytes, and subsequently neutrophilic granulocytes. Together, they release various pro-inflammatory messenger substances and enzymes. As a relevant example, they secrete proteases and disable antiproteases, an imbalance that destabilizes lung tissue. Of particular importance are several cytokines that are significantly elevated in the plasma of patients with COPD signals. In addition to the pathophysiologically clearly defined neutrophilic inflammation, there are also COPD patients with a predominantly eosinophilic inflammation, which could overlap with allergic bronchial asthma. Furthermore, inhaled pollutants can lead to oxidative stress, which increases inflammation and remodeling. Respiratory infections, in most cases bacterial infections, can trigger an exacerbation of already established COPD, in most cases bacterial infections. In addition to conventional medication, in case of refractory therapy, treatment with biologics could be an option.

Keywords: inflammation, macrophages, T-lymphocytes, cytokines, respiratory infection, immunomodulation

1. Introduction

COPD (chronic obstructive pulmonary disease) is a disease of the lungs with permanent narrowing of the bronchial system, resulting from chronic inflammation of the small airways. This obstructive bronchiolitis causes increased mucus production. Lung tissue remodeling occurs and finally fibrosis and destruction of lung tissue lead to pulmonary emphysema. This causes a collapse of the small airways during exhalation. The patients suffer from coughing, massive sputum production, and shortness of breath [1–4].

This book chapter describes the underlying inflammatory processes. The players involved in inflammation are described in more detail, various forms of inflammation or damage are distinguished from one another, and the role of respiratory infections as a trigger is highlighted.

 IntechOpen

2. Players involved in inflammation

Leukocytes as macrophages, T-lymphocytes, and neutrophilic granulocytes are involved in the inflammation processes in COPD. These cells can be activated by pollutants, such as cigarette smoke or fine dust, and by infections [5–7].

Macrophages have the following functions: As M1 macrophages, they promote inflammatory reactions by secreting cytokines, such as IL-6 (interleukin-6) or TNF- α (tumor necrosis factor-α), at the site of inflammation. In this way, they initiate and regulate the body's defense reactions. They phagocytize foreign cells. They act as professional antigen-presenting cells by presenting antigen fragments coupled to MHC (major histocompatibility complex) class II proteins to adaptive immunity cells. They remove cellular debris via phagocytosis. As M2 macrophages, they promote the healing process of inflammation (inflammatory resolution) and secrete messenger substances with an anti-inflammatory effect. As a result, they support wound healing, among other things. The mobilization of leukocytes from the blood and their migration to the site of infection in peripheral tissues is a major step in innate immunity. Macrophages make up only about 10% of all macrophages in the bronchial secretion of healthy people, but up to 90% in the secretion of people with COPD. But in macrophages of patients with COPD, the clearance of the bacteria is decreased. These macrophages also show a defective clearance of apoptotic cells, leading to accumulation of necrotic material in the lungs, causing chronic inflammation. The accumulation of these inflammatory macrophages in the lung seems to be supported by an epigenetic factor called PRMT7 (protein arginine methyltransferase7). In people with COPD, PRMT7 is increased in the progenitor cells from which the macrophages develop. The number of macrophages and thus the severity of COPD are related to the increased PRMT7 values in the lung tissue. Investigated in a mouse model, the animals do not develop COPD when the production of PRMT7 is inhibited. In future, PRMT7 could be a suitable target for future therapeutic or even preventive approaches to COPD in humans [4–7].

T-lymphocytes are divided into two main groups, which differ in their function and the expression of their surface molecules CD4 or CD8: CD4+ T cells differentiate into helper cells or regulatory cells (Tregs) and induce or inhibit other immune cells. Naive CD4+ T cells can be stimulated through direct contact with antigen-presenting cells, such as dendritic cells. Tregs inhibit autoimmune processes and can suppress increased inflammation. Depending on the surrounding cytokine milieus, they can be divided into different subgroups, which have distinct immunomodulatory effector functions. The two most obvious subgroups are the natural Tregs and the inducible or adaptive ones. The natural Tregs leave the thymus as an effector cell and are essential for the formation of self-tolerance, whereas the inducible Tregs develop in the periphery and are activated by exogenous antigens. Tregs transmit their suppressive effects on other T cells or antigen-presenting dendritic cells via contact-dependent mechanisms. Smokers with COPD and emphysema have significantly less Tregs in the lungs, in comparison to control groups (smokers without COPD and healthy nonsmokers). The CD8+ T cells are in front, especially effector cells of the adaptive immune system. After the primary activation, the CD8+ T cells start their proliferation and differentiation into a cytotoxic effector cell. Its key role is to control inflammation by targeting infected cells [4–7].

Neutrophilic granulocytes are recruited to the inflamed areas in the lung, where they become activated and thereby their inflammatory mediators. Increased numbers of activated neutrophils are found in the sputum and bronchoalveolar lavage fluid of patients with COPD and correlate with disease severity, although few neutrophils are seen in the airway wall and lung parenchyma, reflecting their rapid transit through these tissues. Smoking has a direct stimulating effect on neutrophilic granulocyte production and release. Recruitment of neutrophilic granulocytes to the airways involves initial adhesion to endothelial cells through E-selectin, which is up-regulated on endothelial cells in the airways of patients with COPD. Activated neutrophilic granulocytes also release proteolytic enzymes, such as the neutrophil elastase, cathepsin G, and proteinase-3, leading to a proteinase/antiproteinase imbalance. Neutrophil elastase leads to proteolysis in the lungs and degrades many components of the extracellular matrix [4–8].

Dendritic cells are a link between innate and adaptive immunity. The respiratory system contains a network of dendritic cells localized near the surface, and they are ideally located to signal the entry of inhaled foreign substances. Dendritic cells can activate a variety of other immune cells, including macrophages, T-lymphocytes, and neutrophilic granulocytes, and therefore dendritic cells play a significant role in the pulmonary response to cigarette smoke and other inhaled noxious agents. Dendritic cells are activated in the lungs of patients with COPD and are linked to disease severity [5–7].

Cytokines, which are produced and secreted among others by T-lymphocytes, function as players in the humoral system and form together with the cellular system a generalized orchestra of immune response. In several studies, the expression of cytokines was measured in patients with COPD compared with healthy persons. Furthermore, in the population of COPD patients, the correlation between cytokine expression and clinical characteristics or severity was investigated. As result, significant correlations were found in the way that in the plasma of COPD patients, elevated levels of cytokines were identified compared to healthy controls. But there is a large variation between different studies with contradicting results. A selection of the probably most relevant cytokines is briefly presented below [6, 7, 9].

IL-1ß is produced by activated macrophages and plays a role in apoptosis as well as in cell proliferation and differentiation. It is involved in the development of chronic inflammatory diseases, such as COPD. IL-1ß activates macrophages from patients with COPD to secrete inflammatory cytokines, chemokines, and matrix metalloproteinase. There is an increase in the concentration of IL-1ß in sputum of COPD, which is correlated with disease severity [6, 7, 9–12].

IL-2 is also called T-cell growth factor because it stimulates the proliferation and differentiation of T and B lymphocytes. Additionally, it stimulates the production of various other interleukins, INF-γ (interferon-γ) and TNF-α. Cytotoxic cells, such as natural killer cells, lymphokine-activated killer cells, and tumor-infiltrating lymphocytes, which also express the IL-2 receptor, are activated as well [6, 7, 11, 13].

IL-5 is produced by Th2 lymphocytes and in high expression in COPD patients. It seems feasible to inhibit IL-5 to achieve suppression of inflammatory and oxidative stress responses. There is a close association between IL-5 and the aggregation and differentiation of eosinophil. Sputum levels of IL-5 in patients with stable COPD correlate with the degree of eosinophilia [6, 7, 10, 12, 14–16].

IL-6 binds to specific membrane-bound IL-6 receptors found exclusively on hepatocytes and leukocytes. These receptors initiate an intracellular signaling cascade via the membrane-bound gp130 (glycoprotein 130), which is found on the cell membranes of many cell types and leads to trans-signaling cascades. In addition, IL-6 binds to the soluble IL-6 receptor. This complex also binds to the glycoprotein 130. The activation of glycoprotein 130 causes the phosphorylation of JAK (Janus-activated kinase), leading to the activation of several signaling pathways important for the immune response. The activated MAP (mitogen-activated protein) kinase pathway and the likewise activated JAK-STAT (signal transducers and activators of transcription) signaling pathway lead to the intra-cellular transcription of specific target genes relevant to the immune response. This process characterizes interleukin-6 as a lymphocyte-stimulating factor or as an activator of acute-phase proteins. Furthermore, IL-6 participates in the regulation of leukocyte apoptosis, namely with proapoptotic and antiapoptotic active components. In the case of activated T-lymphocytes, the soluble IL-6 receptor is necessary for mediating these effects because activated T-lymphocytes usually have no membrane-bound IL-6 receptors [6, 7, 9–13].

IL-8 is also known as a neutrophilic chemotactic factor. It can be secreted by any cells with toll-like receptors that engage in the innate immune response. As a local inflammatory mediator, it mobilizes neutrophilic granulocytes through chemotactic stimuli and supports their degranulation. In addition to stimulating neutrophilic granulocytes, interleukin-8 also recruits basophilic granulocytes and T-lymphocytes. IL-8 also stimulates phagocytosis. In its target cells, IL-8 can increase intracellular Ca^{2+} and the respiratory burst, which means the release of reactive oxygen species by macrophages and neutrophilic granulocytes during phagocytosis [6, 7, 11–13, 15].

IL-10 is mainly secreted by monocytes and T-lymphocytes. It plays a significant role in modulating inflammatory processes by preventing an excessive immune response. It is one of the most important anti-inflammatory cytokines and is important for the development of immune tolerance. It directs the T-lymphocyte response more from T-helper cell Th1 to Th2. The anti-inflammatory effects include the inhibition of activated macrophages, which produce IL-10 themselves as a negative feedback regulation. Furthermore, they include the inhibition of the production of pro-inflammatory factors, such as IFN-γ, TNF-α, and other cytokines. The ability of monocytes to present antigens is suppressed. They are stimulated more by phagocytosis. However, dendritic cells that have already differentiated are not inhibited by IL-10 because they no longer have an IL-10 receptor [5–7, 9, 12, 13].

IL-12 is produced by activated macrophages, dendritic cells, and airway epithelial cells. It plays a vital role in differentiating and activating Th1 cells, particularly in the production of IFN-γ. By influencing the cell's own defense mechanisms in this way, IL-12 also influences the intensity and duration of intracellular infections [6, 7, 9, 11].

IL-13 is produced among others by Th2 helper cells and stimulates the differentiation of B-lymphocytes. It is involved as a messenger in processes of the immune system, especially in triggering allergic reactions. IL-13 is a relevant mediator for triggering asthma attacks. IL-13 induces matrix metalloproteinases in the airways. These enzymes are required to induce the aggression of inflammatory cells into the airways. IL-13 can also induce collagen expression by fibroblasts [3, 6, 7, 12, 13].

IL-17 family contains six isoforms. IL-17A signaling drives several effector functions, including chemokine induction, cell infiltration, antimicrobial peptide production, tissue barrier function, and remodeling. The levels of IL-17A, the predominant cytokine of Th17 cells, are increased in the sputum of COPD patients. Furthermore, increased Th17 cells can be detected in bronchial biopsies of COPD patients. IL-17B is a pro-inflammatory mediator that accelerates neutrophil recruitment and migration, and it attenuates mucosal inflammation. IL-17C is known to be important for host defense against pathogens such as pseudomonas aeruginosa. IL-17D triggers the secretion of several inflammatory cytokines, such as IL-6 and IL-8. IL-17E-mediated responses depend on the airway epithelium, mast cells, eosinophils, and Th2 cells, thereby contributing to the immunopathogenesis of asthma. IL-17F plays a critical role in inflammatory responses and mucosal barrier maintenance, and it plays a central role in allergic airway diseases [6, 7, 9, 10, 12, 13].

IL-18 is produced by a variety of cells, including macrophages and dendritic cells. Together with interleukin-12, it induces (in cooperation with IL-12) the cell-mediated immune defense after a confrontation with microbial lipopolysaccharides. When stimulated with IL-18, natural killer cells and certain T cells secrete IFN-γ and type II interferon, which play an important role in stimulating macrophages [6, 7, 9, 10, 12].

IL-23 is an inflammatory cytokine, which plays a key role in regulating Th17 cells, and there is an increased expression in the bronchial mucosa of patients with COPD [6, 7, 10, 11].

IL-32 is secreted by T-lymphocytes, natural killer cells, and monocytes. L-32 acts as a regulator of innate and adaptive immune responses and has been confirmed to participate in the inflammatory process of COPD as a proinflammatory factor. While IL-32 induces next to other cytokines TNF-α, its depletion reduces IFN-γ production, suggesting a regulatory feedback mechanism. IL-32 is highly expressed in the lung tissue of patients with COPD, and alveolar wall and bronchial epithelial cells are the main expression sites. There is a strong positive correlation between serum IL-32 concentration and GOLD (global initiative for obstructive lung disease) score, which suggested that IL-32 might be a molecular biomarker that reflects the severity of COPD [6, 7, 9].

IL-33 is a cytokine belonging to the IL-1 superfamily that also includes IL-1α, IL-1β, and IL-18. IL-33 induces T-lymphocytes and other leukocytes, such as mast cells, eosinophilic, and basophilic granulocytes, to produce type 2 cytokines. IL-33 has been associated with inflammatory diseases, such as bronchial asthma and allergy. It could also be of importance in COPD. Previous studies have shown that the IL-33 level in the blood is increased during acute exacerbations of COPD [6, 7, 10, 16, 17].

INF-γ is formed by T-lymphocytes after contact with antigen-presenting macrophages and is characterized by its immune-stimulating, especially antiviral and antitumor effects. An important task of INF-γ is the activation of macrophages and thus the stimulation and support of the cellular defense. It promotes the production of bactericidal substances, such as nitric oxide and reactive oxygen species, by the macrophages and optimizes the process of fusion of phagosomes with lysosomes inside the macrophage. One importance of IFN-γ in the immune system is its ability to inhibit viral replication directly. Aberrant IFN-γ expression is associated with some autoinflammatory and autoimmune diseases [6, 7, 9, 11, 12].

TGF-ß (transforming growth factor-ß) induces the proliferation of fibroblasts and airway smooth muscle cells. It is generated from a latent precursor through oxidative stress and various proteases. TGF-ß regulates the proliferation, differentiation, apoptosis, and adhesion of cells. The expression is increased by airway epithelial cells and macrophages from small airways of patients with COPD [6, 7, 9].

TNF-α is produced mainly by macrophages, which are stimulated to phagocytosis. In the liver, the formation of acute phase proteins, such as CRP, is stimulated. TNF-α promotes a local inflammatory response in foreign stimuli or bacterial infections. Furthermore, TNF-α polymorphism may play an important role in COPD susceptibility. TNF-α stimulates and activates the transcription factor NF-κB (nuclear factor "kappa-light-chain-enhancer" of activated B-cells), which occurs in every human cell, but mainly in B-lymphocytes. NF-κB is of immense importance in the regulation of the immune response, cell proliferation, and apoptosis. NF-κB act as a principal component for several common respiratory illnesses, such as COPD [5–7, 9–13, 15, 18].

TSLP (thymic stromal lymphopoietin) is a cytokine belonging to the IL-7 family. It is increased in the airway epithelium of patients with COPD. Under certain pathological conditions, increased formation of TSLP can occur. TSLP can be released as a danger signal to allergens or microorganisms. The result is increased activation of dendritic cells, which causes Th2 cells to mature. Furthermore, TSLP causes activation of macrophages, which produce chemokines that attract neutrophilic and eosinophilic granulocytes and mast cells [6, 7, 9, 10, 16].

GM-CSF (granulocyte-macrophage colony-stimulating factor) is part of the immune response to antigens and mitogens. It owes its name to its ability to stimulate the differentiation of hematopoietic stem cells in the bone marrow into macrophages and granulocytes. It is released by alveolar macrophages of patients with COPD and is involved in the differentiation and survival of macrophages and neutrophilic granulocytes [6, 7, 9, 11, 12].

3. Forms of inflammation or damage

Neutrophilic inflammation can be induced by cigarette smoke, fine dust, bacteria, and viruses, resulting in the release of neutrophilic mediators, including IL-8, which signal through its receptor on neutrophils. Macrophages are activated as well, and attract Th17 cells to release IL-17, which stimulates the release of IL-6 and IL-8 from epithelial cells. Neutrophils are maintained in the airway by TNF-α and GM-CSF (granulocyte-macrophage colony-stimulating factor) and release neutrophil elastase. Neutrophils also generate oxidative stress, which further activates inflammation and induces corticosteroid resistance. The neutrophilic inflammation in COPD is unresponsive to corticosteroids, even in high doses. Other therapies directed toward neutrophilic inflammation, including antibodies against TNF-α, have been largely clinically ineffective as well. A CXCR2 (chemokine receptor-2) antagonist, which blocks the chemotactic effect of IL-8 and related chemokines, is at least able to reduce the neutrophils in the sputum of COPD patients but has no clinical benefit on lung function, symptoms, or exacerbations. Neutrophil elastase is a major proteinase in primary granules in neutrophils that participates in the microbicidal activity. It induces airway remodeling with increased mucin secretion and impaired ciliary motility, it interrupts epithelial repair by promoting cellular apoptosis, and it activates inflammation by increasing cytokine expression [1, 4–8, 14].

Eosinophilic inflammation is well-known in patients with bronchial asthma. Some people have clinical features from both diseases, bronchial asthma and COPD. In case of such overlap, airway epithelial cells can release the upstream cytokines TSLP and IL-33 in response to cigarette smoke and virus infection, which recruit Th2 and type 2 innate lymphoid cells, which secrete IL-5, resulting in eosinophilic inflammation. Eosinophils may be attracted into the lungs by CCL5 (chemokine (C-C motif) ligand) and maintained in the lungs by IL-5 and GM-CSF. Patients with so-called eosinophilic COPD may have a better response to corticosteroid therapy and more reversibility to bronchodilators, and these patients show an increase in sputum eosinophils and an increased FeNO, which are characteristic features of asthma [1, 5–7, 14].

Protease-antiprotease imbalance means that inhaled pollutants, such as cigarette smoke and fine dust, activate immune cells like macrophages and T-helper cells, which release inflammatory messengers. These signals cause neutrophilic granulocytes to migrate into the bronchial mucosa. Together with the macrophages, they release cell-damaging proteases. And at the same time, protective antiprotease is disabled. According to current knowledge, this imbalance of proteases and antiproteases favors the formation of pulmonary emphysema. Various proteases produced by inflammatory cells and epithelial cells are elevated in many people with COPD [3, 19].

Oxidant-antioxidant imbalance leads to inflammatory reactions due to oxidative stress. As a result, pulmonary cells are damaged, and inflammation is further promoted. This accelerates the development of COPD or emphysema. Oxidative stress also increases mucus production, the formation of proteases, and the migration of neutrophilic granulocytes into the bronchial mucosa. An oxidant-antioxidant imbalance also occurs in other lung diseases, such as pulmonary fibrosis or bronchial asthma [3, 5, 15, 19].

Apoptosis is critical for the maintenance of normal tissue homeostasis and is in equilibrium with proliferation and differentiation. There is increasing evidence that disturbance of the balance between apoptosis and proliferation in lung tissue contributes to the pathogenesis of COPD. Several experimental studies in animal models of COPD provide more insight into the association between cigarette smoking, apoptosis, and the development of emphysema. Epithelial cells in the small airways express TGF-β, which then induces local fibrosis. VEGF (vascular endothelial growth factor) appears to be necessary to maintain alveolar cell integrity, and blockade of VEGF receptors in rats induces apoptosis of alveolar cells and an emphysema-like pathology [19].

4. Infections and inflammation

Epidemiological studies point to a connection between respiratory infections in the past and the incidence of COPD. For example, viral pneumonia in childhood increases the risk for the later development of COPD. With an already existing COPD, acute respiratory infections can trigger an exacerbation. In most cases, bacterial infections cause a trigger. Streptococcus pneumoniae, haemophilus influenzae, moraxella catarrhalis, and pseudomonas aeruginosa have been identified to act as triggers, also tuberculosis can cause an exacerbation of COPD. Furthermore, fungi are potential triggers as well. Viruses have not been found to be common triggers; exceptions are rhinoviruses and SARS-CoV-2 [7].

Patients with underlying COPD are vulnerable to COVID-19, and in fact, COPD is one of the high-risk factors for severe illness associated with COVID-19. This may be related to poor underlying lung reserves and increased expression of ACE-2 (angiotensin-converting enzyme-2) receptor in small airways. One research group established an airway epithelium model to study SARS-CoV-2 infection in healthy and COPD lung cells. They found that both the entry receptor ACE2 and the cofactor transmembrane protease TMPRSS2 are expressed at higher levels on non-ciliated goblet cell, a novel target for SARS-CoV-2 infection. They observed that SARS-CoV-2 induced due to an infection of goblet cells syncytium formation and cell sloughing. They also found that SARS-CoV-2 replication is increased in the COPD airway epithelium, likely due to COPD-associated goblet cell hyperplasia [20–22].

5. Use of biologics in refractory therapy of COPD

Drug therapy of COPD includes various pharmaceuticals, some of which are inhaled and some orally used, in various combinations. These include muscarinic antagonists, ß2-sympathomimetics, corticosteroids, mucolytics, antitussives, beta-blocker, N-acetyl-L-cysteine, antibiotics, oxygen, and vaccinations against pneumococcus infection, pertussis, influenza, and COVID-19. The administration of the phosphodiesterase-4 inhibitor roflumilast is possible as add-on therapy in patients with COPD who repeatedly exacerbate despite therapy, who are assigned to the chronic bronchitis phenotype, and who have an FEV1 (forced expiratory pressure in 1 s) <50% [2, 3, 15].

Furthermore, there are several biologics which could be used in the case of refractory therapy of COPD, especially if there is a combination with bronchial asthma. The following shows a representative selection of biologics, which are mostly used in the treatment of other inflammatory diseases, but which can be considered in individual cases of COPD in particularly severe courses that are resistant to conventional treatment options:

- **Benralizumab** (*Fasenra*®) is a humanized monoclonal antibody that binds with high affinity and specificity to the IL-5 receptor. This receptor is localized on the surface of eosinophilic granulocytes. Apoptosis of the granulocytes occurs and leads to a reduction in the inflammatory reaction. Benralizumab is a potential add-on therapy in adult patients with severe eosinophilic COPD as well as bronchial asthma. Application of benralizumab is subcutaneous injection [1, 6, 15, 16].

- **Brodalumab** (*Kyntheum*®) is a recombinant human monoclonal antibody. It binds selectively to subunit A of the IL-17 receptor. This blocks the activity of IL-17A and IL-17F and inhibits the inflammatory process. It is used to treat psoriasis. Brodalumab is given as a subcutaneous injection [6, 23].

- **Canakinumab** (*Ilaris*®) is a human monoclonal antibody that inhibits the activity of IL-1β, thereby inhibiting the inflammatory processes. Canakinumab is indicated for the treatment of periodic fever syndromes, familial Mediterranean fever, systemic juvenile idiopathic arthritis, and gouty arthritis. Canakinumab is administered subcutaneously [1, 6].

- **Dupilumab** (*Dupixent*®) is a humanized monoclonal antibody that binds to the alpha subunit of the IL-4 receptor, blocking IL-4 and IL-13 signaling. The antibody had shown good efficacy in patients with bronchial asthma and elevated eosinophils. Furthermore, in severe atopic dermatitis and rhinosinusitis dupilumab may help as well. In therapy-refractory COPD, the use of dupilumab can be considered. Application is by subcutaneous injection [6, 16, 23].

- **Etanercept** (*Enbrel*®) is a selective immunosuppressive and anti-inflammatory drug from the group of TNF-α inhibitors. It is a dimeric fusion protein composed of the extracellular ligand-binding domain of TNF receptor-2 and the Fc (fragment crystallizable) domain of human IgG1 (immunoglobulin G1). It binds to TNF-α and blocks its effects. Etanercept is used in the therapy of psoriasis and rheumatic diseases. The solution for injection is administered subcutaneously [1, 6, 15].

- **Infliximab** (*Remicade*®) is a chimeric monoclonal antibody against TNF-α and blocks its inflammatory effects. Infliximab is used as an immunosuppressant. Main indications for therapy are Crohn's disease and rheumatoid arthritis. In the case of severe and therapy-resistant COPD, the administration of infliximab may be an option. The medicine is given as an intravenous infusion [1, 6, 15].

- **Mepolizumab** (*Nucala*®) is a humanized monoclonal antibody against IL-5 and inhibits the binding of IL-5 to its receptor on the cell surface of eosinophils. Some authors regard therapy with mepolizumab as a therapeutic advance for a subgroup of patients with severe eosinophilic COPD or bronchial asthma. Mepolizumab is given as a solution for subcutaneous injection [1, 6, 15, 16].

- **Omalizumab** (*Xolair*®) is a humanized monoclonal antibody against IgE and thereby suppresses an allergic reaction. It is used therapeutically in the fourth step of asthma step therapy for severe allergic bronchial asthma, and in chronic spontaneous urticaria, if the conventional therapy does not improve the disease properly. In the case of COPD and allergic bronchial asthma overlap, omalizumab may be helpful. It is injected subcutaneously [6, 16, 23].

- **Reslizumab** (*Cinqaero* ®) is a humanized monoclonal antibody against IL-5 and reduces the number of eosinophils, which leads to lower inflammatory activity. Reslizumab is available as a concentrate solution for intravenous infusion [6, 16].

- **Secukinumab** (*Cosentyx* ®) is a recombinant human monoclonal antibody that acts by selectively binding to IL-17A and blocks its interaction with the IL-17 receptor, preventing the release of proinflammatory cytokines. It is mainly used in psoriasis. Secukinumab is administered subcutaneously [6, 23].

- **Tezepelumab** (*Tezspirie* ®) is a monoclonal antibody from the group of TSLP inhibitors. The effects are based on binding to TSLP, which inhibits interaction with its receptor. Tezepelumab is approved for adjunctive maintenance therapy for the relief of severe, uncontrolled bronchial asthma. The solution for injection is given subcutaneously [6, 23].

Other biologics are currently in clinical trials and will be launched in near future. An example is itepekimab, which is under investigation in a phase 3 study. In a current study, the researchers first carried out genetic investigations to determine whether genetic variants within the IL-33 signaling pathways are associated with the risk of COPD. They found that genetic variants that resulted in loss of IL-33 function reduced the risk of COPD. Variants that caused IL-33 to be more active increased the risk of COPD. In addition, they examined the safety and effectiveness of the IL-33-antibody itepekimab in moderate to severe COPD. Itepekimab targets IL-33, thereby inhibiting the activity of the protein. 343 patients between the ages of 40 and 75 were included in the study. All were current or former smokers with a COPD diagnosis of at least 1 year. They were randomly assigned either to the itepekimab or placebo group. In addition to standard therapy, people in the itepekimab group received the antibody as injections every 2 weeks. The other group received a drug-free placebo instead of the antibody. The effect of itepekimab on the annual rate of acute COPD exacerbations and lung function was analyzed. When both groups were compared, there were initially no significant differences. However, a subgroup analysis found that itepekimab significantly reduced exacerbation rates and improved lung function in ex-smokers with COPD. The positive effects also persisted during the 20-week follow-up period after treatment. The side effects were about the same in both groups. According to the researchers, the study does not show any advantage of itepekimab for current smokers with COPD. However, for ex-smokers with COPD, this biological therapy could be an option to improve the rate of disease worsening and lung function. Future studies should therefore focus even more on this subgroup of patients. Two-phase three clinical trials are already underway to confirm and better understand the potential of the novel therapy in ex-smokers with COPD [3, 6, 23, 24].

Author details

Christian Peiser
Charité—Medical University Berlin, Germany

*Address all correspondence to: christian.peiser@charite.de

References

[1] Brightling C, Greening N. Airway inflammation in COPD: Progress to precision medicine. The European Respiratory Journal. 2019;**53**:1802460

[2] BÄK B, KBV KB. Arbeitsgemeinschaft der Wissenschaftlichen Medizinischen Fachgesellschaften (AWMF). Nationale Versorgungsleitlinie COPD – Kurzfassung. 2021. Available from: www.leitlinien.de/copd

[3] München HZ. Deutsches Forschungszentrum für Gesundheit und Umwelt. Lungeninformationsdienst. 2022. Available from: www.lungeninformationsdienst.de/krankheiten/copd

[4] Wang Y, Xu J, Meng Y, Adcock IM, Yao X. Role of inflammatory cells in airway remodeling in COPD. International Journal of Chronic Obstructive Pulmonary Disease. 2018;**13**:3341-3348

[5] Barnes PJ. Inflammatory mechanisms in patients with chronic obstructive pulmonary disease. The Journal of Allergy and Clinical Immunology. 2016;**138**:16-27

[6] DocCheck Community GmbH. DocCheck Flexikon. Available from: https://flexikon.doccheck.com

[7] Wikimedia Foundation Inc. Wikipedia – Die freie Enzyklopädie. Available from: https://de.wikipedia.org

[8] Voynow JA, Shinbashi M. Neutrophil elastase and chronic lung disease. Biomolecules. 2021;**11**:1065

[9] Barnes PJ. The cytokine network in chronic obstructive pulmonary disease. American Journal of Respiratory Cell and Molecular Biology. 2009;**41**:631-638

[10] Caramori G, Adcock IM, Stefano A, Chung KF. Cytokine inhibition in the treatment of COPD. International Journal of Chronic Obstructive Pulmonary Disease. 2014;**9**:297-412

[11] Morello Gearhart A, Cavallazzi R, Peyrani P, Wiemken TL, Furmanek SP, Reyes-Vega A, et al. Lung cytokines and systemic inflammation in patients with COPD. The University of Louisville Journal of Respiratory Infections. 2017;**1**(4):4

[12] Obling N, Backer V, Hurst JR, Bodtger U. Nasal and systemic inflammation in chronic obstructive pulmonary disease (COPD). Respiratory Medicine. 2022;**195**:106774

[13] Uzeloto JS, de Toledo-Arruda AC, Silva BSA, Golim MA, Braz AMM, de Lima FF, et al. Systemic cytokine profiles of CD4+ T lymphocytes correlate with clinical features and functional status in stable COPD. International Journal of Chronic Obstructive Pulmonary Disease. 2020;**15**:2931-2940

[14] Barnes PJ. Inflammatory endotypes in COPD. Allergy. 2019;**74**:1249-1256

[15] Guo P, Li R, Piao TH, Wang CL, Wu XL, Cai HY. Pathological mechanism and targeted drugs of COPD. International Journal of Chronic Obstructive Pulmonary Disease. 2022;**17**:1565-1575

[16] Kusumozo M, Mathis BJ. Biologic treatments for asthma and chronic obstructive pulmonary disorder. Allergie. 2021;**1**:92-107

[17] Chan BCL, Lam CWK, Tam LS, Wong CK. IL33: Roles in allergic inflammation and therapeutic

perspectives. Frontiers in Immunology. 2019;**10**:364

[18] Alharbi KS, Fuloria NK, Fuloria S, Rahman SB, Al-Malki WH, Javed Shaikh MA, et al. Nuclear factor-kappa B and its role in inflammatory lung disease. Chemico-Biological Interactions. 2021;**345**:109568

[19] Demedts IK, Demoor T, Bracke KR, Joos GF, Brusselle GG. Role of apoptosis in the pathogenesis of COPD and pulmonary emphysema. Respiratory Research. 2006;**7**:53

[20] Leung JM, Niikura M, Yang CWT, Sin DD. COVID-19 and COPD. The European Respiratory Journal. 2020;**56**:2002108

[21] Osan JK, Talukdar SN, Feldmann F, Ann DeMontigny B, Jerome K, Bailey KL, et al. Goblet cell hyperplasia increases SARS-CoV-2 infection in COPD. bioRxiv. 2020;**11**(11):379099. DOI: 10.1101/2020.11.11.379099

[22] Sin DD. COVID-19 in COPD: A growing concern. E Clinical Medicine. 2020;**26**:100546

[23] Cazzola M, Matera MG, Calzetta L, Rogliani P. Biologics in asthma and chronic obstructive pulmonary disorder. Respiratory Pulmonary Disease. 2022;**7**:8-14

[24] Rabe KF, Celli BR, Wechsler ME, Abdulai RM, Luo X, Boomsma MM, et al. Safety and efficacy of itepekimab in patients with moderate-to-severe COPD: A genetic association study and randomised, double-blind, phase 2a trial. The Lancet Respiratory Medicine. 2021;**9**:1288-1298

Chapter 4

The Risk Factors of Frequent Exacerbations of COPD

Aigoul Zinnatullina and Rustem Khamitov

Abstract

We wanted to identify risk factors for re-hospitalization of patients with exacerbation and to assess the quality of medical care in outpatient and inpatient settings. Analysis of medical records of patients with exacerbation of chronic obstructive pulmonary disease treated in hospitals 2015–2018 years. Risk factors for repeated hospitalizations were identified as male (relative risk 3.49; 95% confidence interval 1.45–8.43; $p < 0.05$), age over 70 years ($p < 0.05$), smoking experience >40 years ($p < 0.05$), COPD duration >10 years (relative risk 3.48; 95% confidence interval 2.27–5.34; $p < 0.05$), the presence of three or more comorbid pathologies (relative risk 2.0; 95% confidence interval 1.23–3.4; $p < 0.05$). Also important is the form of non-compliance with the regime in outpatient conditions and concomitant diseases in the hospital. Most of the factors are unmodifiable, so it is important to optimize treatment and control patient adherence. It is necessary to pay more attention to non-drug treatment methods: maintaining physical activity and quitting smoking. Taking into account the identified shortcomings in the quality of medical care provided to patients, they indicate the need for more active implementation of guidelines on chronic obstructive pulmonary disease in real clinical practice.

Keywords: chronic obstructive pulmonary disease, readmission, risk factors, exacerbations, COPD

1. Introduction

Chronic obstructive pulmonary disease (COPD) is an urgent problem of modern pulmonology. Currently, COPD is in third place on the list of causes of death in the world and mortality from it continues to grow [1]. The main cause of death in patients with COPD is the progression of the underlying disease, which is most often caused by frequent severe exacerbations. Exacerbations of COPD negatively affect the patient's quality of life, worsen symptoms, and accelerate the rate of decline in lung function, and are associated with significant mortality [2]. About 50–80% of COPD patients die from respiratory causes [3]. So, comorbid pathology is an integral feature of COPD, and 50% of the causes of fatal cases are "extrapulmonary" [4].

1.1 Goal

Identification of risk factors for repeated hospitalizations associated with exacerbation of the chronic obstructive pulmonary disease, followed by an assessment of the quality of care provided to patients at the outpatient and hospital stages.

2. Material and methods

A retrospective analysis of medical records of inpatient patients with acute COPD who were admitted to the therapeutic department of one of the multidisciplinary hospitals in Kazan from January 1, 2015 to December 31, 2018 was conducted.

Statistical data processing was performed using the SPSS Statistical programs. The data obtained are presented in the form of M ± σ and in the form of frequency (for absolute values). To assess the significance of differences, Pearson's *t*-test method was used. The differences were considered significant at $p < 0.05$. To assess the risk factors for frequent hospitalizations, we calculated absolute and relative risk (RR) with a 95% confidence interval (CI) at $p < 0.05$.

3. Results and discussion

During the study period, 423 patients were admitted to the therapeutic department for COPD exacerbation. Of these, 276 were hospitalized once in a calendar year (control group), and 147 cases of hospitalization occurred in 60 patients who were hospitalized 2 or more times in a year (38 patients (63.33%)—2 times, 17 (28.33%)—3 times, 5 (8.33%)—4 times in a calendar year). Thus, 14.2% of patients required repeated hospitalizations due to an exacerbation of the disease (the main group). Men prevailed among the single-time hospitalized patients with a male/female ratio of 2.6:1, and among thex re-hospitalized patients with a ratio of 11:1. Belonging to the male sex increased the risk of repeated hospitalizations by 3.5 times (RR 3.49; 95% DI 1.45–8, 43). The mean age of patients in the control group was 69.49 ± 0.64 years (men: 67.68 ± 0.75 years, women: 74.28 ± 1.1 years). The average age of patients in the main group was 70.48 ± 1.22 years (men: 69.53 ± 1.24 years, women: 81 ± 1.84 years). ($p>0.05$). It was found that the age over 70 years increases the risk of repeated hospitalizations by 1.2 times (RR 1.21; 95% CI 0.74–1.86). The average bedtime in the control group was 8.98 ± 0.22 days, and in the main group—9.3 ± 0.33 days ($p < 0.05$). In the main group, the average bed-day in the first hospitalization was 9.32 ± 0.45 days, in the second—9.02 ± 0.6 days, in the third—9.9 ± 0.78 days, and in the fourth—10.2 ± 2.71 days (the number of bed-days during repeated hospitalizations in the main group did not distinguish, $p > 0.05$). There is a tendency to increase the duration of hospitalization, which may be associated with an increase in the severity of the condition of patients requiring repeated hospitalizations during the year.

Unfortunately, not all medical records contained data on the duration of the disease. Information about the duration of COPD was indicated only in 60.66% of cases in the control group. It was found that the average duration of the disease in patients in the control group was 8.51 ± 0.77 years. About 33.7% (93) of patients hospitalized once, were diagnosed with COPD for the first time, while 15 out of 93 patients had a history of chronic bronchitis. Data on the duration of COPD in patients hospitalized repeatedly were also available only in 54.42% of medical records. It turned out that the average duration of COPD in the main group was 11.34 ± 1.33 years ($p < 0.05$). Three patients were diagnosed with COPD for the first time in the first of repeated hospitalizations, and before that, they had a history of chronic bronchitis. The duration of COPD for more than 10 years increases the risk of repeated hospitalizations by 3.5 times (HR 3.48, 95% CI 2.27–5.34).

About 16.3% (45) of patients in the control group, as well as 23.33% (14) of patients in the main group, had a history of occupational hazards (working as a miner, welder, painter, bricklayer, grinder, milling machine, etc.), which could have an impact on the increased risk of frequent COPD exacerbations by almost 1.5 times (RR 1.4–3, 95% CI 0.84–2.42).

Medical records did not provide sufficient data on the fact, duration of smoking, and the number of cigarettes smoked. Only in 30.4% (84) of cases was it possible to determine the average smoking experience in "pack-years." In the control group, the average smoking experience was 37.9 ± 1.7 packs/year. Taking into account the possibility of obtaining information about smoking from several medical records of re-hospitalized patients, the average smoking experience was determined at 50% (30). It was 42.2 ± 3.44 packs/year ($p < 0.05$). Smoking duration of 40 years or more increased the risk of repeated hospitalizations by 1.6 times (RR 1.6, 95% CI 0.87–3.0, $p < 0.05$). Among the control group patients, 35.5% (98) and 29.9% (44) of the main group patients continued to smoke at the time of hospitalization. Only 43% (42) of the once-hospitalized patients and 36.36% (16) of the repeatedly hospitalized patients were recommended to quit smoking at discharge. Recommendations for quitting smoking after the first hospitalization were received by 25% of smokers, after the second hospitalization—by 50% of patients, after the third—by 80% of patients, and after the fourth hospitalization—by 100%. Following the recommendations for quitting smoking,3.3% of patients reported that they had quit smoking at the time of their next hospitalization for COPD exacerbation, half of them—after the second hospitalization.

It should be noted that the largest number of hospitalizations of patients in the control group occurred in the winter and spring months, during this period 63% (173) of patients were hospitalized, which is significantly higher than in the summer and autumn months. No such pattern was found in the main group of patients. On the contrary, the number of hospitalizations during the calendar year remained at the same level (**Figure 1**). Based on the data obtained, it can be assumed that the frequency of hospitalizations of patients in the main group may be more affected by the severity of the underlying disease and the general condition of patients.

All hospitalizations for acute COPD were carried out on an emergency basis. Moreover, 51.45% (142) of single-time hospitalized patients were delivered to the hospital by ambulance teams, 28.26% (78) of patients were referred by local therapists, 12.68% (35)—were delivered by ambulance teams from the polyclinic, 7.61% (21)—went to the hospital on their own. Re-hospitalized patients were also significantly more often delivered to the hospital by ambulance teams: 61.67% (37) of patients were admitted to the first hospital, 63.33% (38) to the second, 86.36% (19) to the third, and 80% (4) to the fourth.

At admission to the hospital, the condition of patients in the control group was assessed as severe in 11.59% (32) of cases, and in the main group—in 10.2% (15) of cases ($p < 0.05$). And due to the severity of respiratory failure 11.96% (33) once hospitalized patients were treated in the intensive care unit (ICU). At the same time, 60.6% (20) of them were admitted to the ICU from the emergency room, and 39.4% (13) were admitted to the ICU from the emergency room—they were

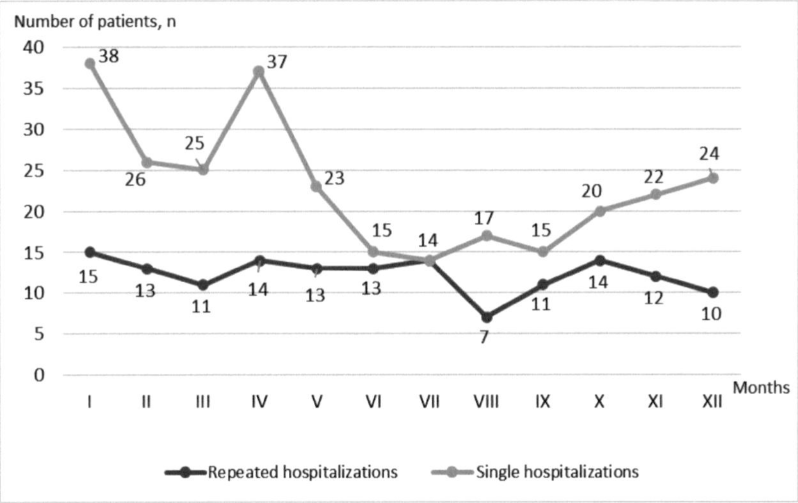

Figure 1.
Dynamics of hospitalizations for exacerbation of chronic obstructive pulmonary disease from January 1, 2015 to December 31, 2018 by month.

transferred from the Department of therapy. Re-admitted patients were admitted to ICU in 10.88% (16) cases, of which 56.25% (9)—were from the emergency room, and 43.75% (7)—were from the therapeutic department. Average bed-day in ICU of patients in the control group was 3.56 ± 0.62 days, and in the main group—4.38 ± 1.39 days ($p < 0.05$). Only 68.75% (22) of patients in the control group and 66.67% (10) of patients in the main group, whose condition was assessed as severe during hospitalization, received intensive care in the intensive care unit.

Mortality in the control group was 3.26%, and in the main group—4.76% ($p < 0.05$). It was found that the proportion of fatal cases among patients hospitalized in ICU from the emergency department, in the control group was 10% (2 out of 20), and in the main group—11.1% (1 out of 9). At the same time, the proportion of deaths among patients transferred to ICU from the therapeutic department was significantly higher in both once-admitted and re-admitted patients and amounted to 53.85% (7 out of 13) and 85.7% (6 out of 7), respectively. The revealed trend may indicate an insufficient assessment of the severity of the patient's condition upon admission to the hospital and untimely provision of intensive care for severe patients, which may be one of the reasons for more frequent deaths in this group of patients.

When evaluating the anamnesis data on outpatient treatment, it was found that 4.4% (8) of patients in the control group did not use inhalers on an outpatient basis, and 19.7% (36) of patients used only emergency medications. Among patients in the main group, 21.3% (23) also did not receive basic therapy ($p < 0.05$). When comparing these recommendations at discharge from the hospital and the history of outpatient therapy during subsequent hospitalization, it was found that 44.6% (29 out of 65) of patients in the main group did not follow the recommendations given to them at discharge. On an outpatient basis, patients were more likely to receive combination therapy with inhaled glucocorticoid steroids (ICS) and long-acting beta-2-agonists (LABA) (31.2% (57) of patients in the control group and 39.8% (43) in the main group), as well as a combination of ICS, LABA and long-acting anticholinergic drugs (13.1% (24) of patients in the control group and 23.1% (25) in the main group).

In none of the cases in the medical records were there data on monitoring the correct inhalation technique and training in the correct use of inhalers, despite the fact that many large studies have shown that training and regular monitoring of inhalation techniques increases the effectiveness of therapy.

As it is known, infectious agents and, in particular, bacteria are not always the cause of COPD exacerbations, so the indications for antibiotic therapy remain rather narrow and include increased shortness of breath, an increase in the amount sputum, and an additional marker confirming the need for antibiotic therapy is an increase in the level of C-reactive protein (CRP) 10 mg/l. In accordance with these recommendations, when patients are admitted to a hospital, it is necessary to conduct a number of laboratory and instrumental research methods to select the correct patient management tactics.

Determination of the C-reactive protein level at admission was performed in 81.5% (225) of cases in the control group. At the same time, in 64% (144) cases, the level of CRP was higher than normal, but in dynamics, the analysis was repeated only in 62.5% (90) of them. It was also found that 10% (5) of patients who underwent CRP analysis only before discharge had elevated levels of C-reactive protein. In the main group of patients, the study of the level of CRP was conducted in 74.2% (109) cases, in half of which (54 cases) it turned out to be higher than normal, but in dynamics only 33.33% (18 out of 54) patients were analyzed. In patients of the main group, the CRP level was determined only before discharge, the indicator was normal. In 13.4% (37) of patients hospitalized once, and y in 21.8% (32) patients who were hospitalized repeatedly the level of C-reactive protein during hospitalization was not determined.

The result of sputum analysis was found in 80% (221) of hospitalizations in the control group, as well as in 83% (122) cases of hospitalizations in the main group. A possible reason for the absence of sputum analysis in 6.5% of patients in the control group and in 3.4% of cases in the main group may be the presence of an unproductive cough.

Bacteriological examination of sputum was performed during hospitalization in 80.4% of patients in the control group, but the result of the study in the medical record was only 9.4% of them. Streptococcus pneumoniae (38.5%), Klebsiella pneumoniae (23%), Pseudomonas aeruginosa (11.5%), Escherichia coli (7.7%), and Haemophilus influenzae (11.5%) were most frequently detected—11.5%. Phlegm bacteriological examination was performed in 76.2% of patients who were hospitalized again, but the result of the study was only in 9.5% of cases. Streptococcus pneumoniae (42.9%), Klebsiella pneumoniae (14.3%), and Pseudomonas aeruginosa (14.3%) were most frequently detected. In more than 90% of cases, etiologically significant growth of microflora was not obtained, which makes it possible to assume inadequate or untimely collection of material for the study.

Hypoxia and subsequent hypoxemia are threatening conditions for the body. One of the most screening diagnostic methods is pulse oximetry [5]. It was revealed that pulse oximetry was performed in the emergency department of the hospital in 81.88% (226) of patients in the control group and 91.8% (135) of patients in the main group. In dynamics, the level of blood oxygen saturation was determined in 82.6% (228) of single-time hospitalized patients and 83.7% (123) re-hospitalized patients.

In the control group, 28.6% (64) of patients had a blood saturation of more than 95%, 45.1% (101) had a saturation of 90–94%, 22.7% (51) had a saturation of 75–89%, and 3.6% (8) had a saturation of less than 75%. In the main group at admission, 21.6% (29) had a blood saturation of more than 95%, 44.1% (59) had a blood saturation of more than 95%. About 90–94%, 32.1% (43)—75–89%, 2.2% (3)—less than 75%.

When analyzing the level of saturation at each subsequent hospitalization separately, it was found that among patients who were hospitalized three times at the time of the first hospitalization, the proportion of patients with blood saturation of more than 95% was 2.25 times higher than at the third hospitalization (23.6% vs. 10.5%). At the same time, there was a tendency to increase in the number of patients with a saturation of 90–94% from the first to the third hospitalization (from 43.6% to 57.9%), as well as with a saturation of 75–89% from the first to the fourth hospitalization (from 30.9% to 60%). There were no significant differences in blood saturation between the first and second hospitalizations.

Spirometry is one of the main methods for determining the degree of air flow restriction, which is necessary for making a diagnosis of COPD and verifying the severity of ventilation disorders. Spirometry is not recommended for acute COPD patients, but it is possible to study the function of external respiration as patients stabilize closer to hospital discharge [3]. Spirometry is especially important for patients who have not previously been diagnosed with COPD, and they accounted for 33.7% (93) patients in the control group and 2% (3) of patients in the main group. When studying medical records it was found that only 38.4% (106) of patients in the control group and 37.4% (55)—the main group, had Spirometry data. Thus, only slightly more than half of the patients in the main group (53.3%) underwent ERF testing in at least one of the hospitalizations. Data were obtained that among single-time hospitalized patients, 10.38% (11) had mild obstructive disorders, 30.2% (32)—medium-heavy, 40.56% (43)—severe, 18.86% (20)—extremely severe. Among the re-hospitalized patients, 28.13% (9) of patients had moderate obstructive disorders, 37.5% (12)—severe, 34.37% (11)—extremely severe. Thus, it was found that the proportion of patients with extremely severe obstructive disorders in the main group was almost twice as high as in the control group.

Chest radiography (CHR) is recommended for all patients with severe COPD to a greater extent for differential diagnosis with other diseases that may be accompanied by increased dyspnea or cough. In accordance with the obtained data , an X-ray examination of the chest was performed in 93.8% (259) of patients in the control group and 84.35% (124) of patients in the main group who were hospitalized. Four patients who were hospitalized once, and three patients who were hospitalized repeatedly were not prescribed radiography of the chest by a general practitioner due to the presence of fluorography results for the last year, which cannot be a reason for refusing the study. It should be noted that all rehospitalized patients underwent radiography of the chest during at least one of their hospitalizations per year.

The revealed defects in laboratory and instrumental diagnostics of patients during COPD exacerbation can lead to underestimation of the severity of the patient's condition, the choice of inadequate management tactics and the amount of therapy.

The main component of COPD treatment in the acute phase is inhaled bronchodilators, the most popular of which are short-acting beta-2-adrenomimetics in possible combination with m-cholinolytics. About 95.65% of patients in the control group and 97.28% of patients in the main group received combined inhaled therapy (fenoterol/ipratropia bromide) via a nebulizer.

According to federal clinical guidelines, the use of systemic glucocorticoids (SCS) during acute disease reduces the time of remission, improves lung function (FEV1), and reduces hypoxemia. It is recommended to use prednisone in a daily dose of 40 mg for 3–5 days with rapid withdrawal of the drug due to the frequent development of side effects, especially in elderly patients. In severe exacerbations of COPD, it is possible to prescribe SGS parenterally [3, 6]. It was found that 65.2% (180) of patients in the control group and 77.55% (114) of patients in the main group received SGS in the hospital. About 61.23% (169) of patients hospitalized once, prednisone was administered parenterally at an average daily dose of 63.55 ± 0.97 mg lasting from 1 to 12 days. At the same time, 14.2% (23) of them were transferred to oral administration of the drug at an average dose of 25 ± 1.5 mg per day for an average of 5.7 ± 0.4 days. Patients of the main group received prednisone parenterally in 74.83% (110) of cases at an average dose of 64.9 ± 2.24 mg/day lasting from 1 to 11 days. About 20.9% (23) of patients after parenteral administration were transferred to oral administration at a dose of 24.35 ± 1.86 mg with an average duration of 5.83 ± 0.52 days. Initially, oral prednisone was administered only in 4% (11) of patients in the control group and in 2.7% (4) of patients in the main group.

It is noted worthy that 12.7% (35) of patients in the control group and 1.4% (2) of patients in the main group did not receive glucocorticoids during hospitalization, which may question the severity of exacerbation and the validity of hospitalization, or be considered a defect in the choice of therapy for COPD exacerbation, which could prolong the time of remission. At the same time, the proportion of patients receiving glucocorticoids both systemically and inhaled was significantly higher: 82.46% (94) of patients in the main group and 55.43% (153) of patients in the control group. At the same time, in 9.78% (27) of cases in the control group and in 6.8% (10) of cases in the main group, when prescribing glucocorticoids, SGS was preferred over inhaled ones, despite the fact that for patients with comorbid pathology budesonide nebulization is a safer alternative to prednisone administration.

Since methylxanthines have a relatively weak bronchodilating effect (compared to beta-2agonists and m-cholinolytics), a small therapeutic range, and pronounced side effects, they are considered second-line drugs in COPD exacerbation and are recommended for patients with poor response to inhaled bronchodilator therapy [7]. However, it was found that theophylline was administered parenterally from the first day in 18.8% of patients in the control group for an average of 4.27 ± 0.29 days, and in 14.3% of patients in the main group—for an average of 4.43 ± 0.37 days. At the same time, 2 patients of the main group a and 2 patients of the control group received theophylline therapy if they had a permanent form of atrial fibrillation.

Oxygen therapy in the hospital was prescribed to patients in the control group only in 21.38% (59) of cases, of which in 11.86% (7) of cases, blood oxygen saturation was more than 95% in air, and in 13.56% (9) of cases, pulse oximetry was not performed. About 29.25% (44) of patients in the main group received oxygen therapy. There were no indications in 11.36% (5) of these cases, and pulse oximetry was not performed in 4.5% (2). At the same time, in the presence of absolute indications, only 56.5% (35) of the medical records of patients in the control group and 54.35% (25) of the main group have data on the appointment of oxygen inhalation.

Based on a comprehensive assessment of the results of the study, in 9.4% (26) of cases in the control group and in 11.5% (17) in the main group, the validity of prescribing antibiotic therapy can be questioned. In 1.8% (5) of cases in the control group and 4.1% (6) of cases in the main group, patients did not receive antibiotics reasonably. In the control group ceftriaxone was prescribed in most cases: in 55% (152) cases—as monotherapy, in 17% (47)—in combination with azithromycin. In all cases of dual antibiotic therapy, community-acquired pneumonia was suspected at the initial examination by a general practitioner, but the diagnosis was confirmed only in 5 out of 47 patients. At the same time, in 10% (25) of cases, an antibiotic replacement was performed, in a third of cases (8) it was not justified according to the medical history. When studying the data of medical records of patients hospitalized repeatedly, it was found that ceftriaxone was prescribed as the starting therapy in 62% of cases, and in 11% of cases (16)—ceftriaxone with azithromycin, of which in a third of cases there was no justification for prescribing dual antibiotic therapy. In almost half of the cases of repeated hospitalization (29 out of 60 patients), patients received the same antibiotic as in the previous one. It was also found that the same antibiotic was prescribed in 38.3% (23) of two consecutive hospitalizations, in 8.3% (5)—three consecutive hospitalizations, and in 1.6% (1)—four times. In addition, it was found that in 9 more cases after ceftriaxone monotherapy, a combination of ceftriaxone with azithromycin or levofloxacin was subsequently prescribed in the previous hospitalization. Thus, we can assume that in 63.3% (38) of cases, when prescribing an antibiotic, therapy in the previous hospitalization was not taken into account.

Comorbidity in COPD plays an important role in its progression and affects the survival of patients with exacerbation of the underlying disease. It was found that patients in the control group had an average of 2.7 ± 0.1 concomitant diseases, and patients in the main group—3.27 ± 0.18. The presence of 3 or more comorbidities increased the risk of repeated hospitalizations by 2 times (RR 2.0; 95% CI 1.23–3.4).

There were no significant differences in the incidence of concomitant diseases such as coronary heart disease (46.6% and 44.6%, respectively) between patients in the main and control groups, diabetes mellitus (13.3% and 12.3%), atrial fibrillation (10% and 10.1%), in 25% and 26.8% of cases, respectively, an increase in pulmonary artery pressure was detected.

COPD itself has significant systemic effects on the body, including weight loss, eating disorders, and skeletal muscle dysfunction. However, it was found that in the control group, the number of patients with body mass deficiency was 2 times higher than in the main group (13.4% vs. 6.7%) ($p < 0.05$). At the same time, the number of overweight and obese patients was the same in both study groups (51.7% and 51.8%). Patients in the main group were significantly more likely to have a history of hypertension (88.3% vs. 72.1%), stage 2 chronic heart failure (CHF 2A) (35% vs. 23.5%), and gastroesophageal reflux disease (GERD) (23.3% vs. 5.8%). When analyzing the data, it was found that the presence of hypertension increased the risk of repeated hospitalizations by 3.5 times (RR 3.55, 95% CI 1.47–8.57, $p < 0.05$), the presence of CHF stage 2A—by 1.5 times (RR 1.5–6, 95% CI 0.98–2, -8–2.5, $p < 0.05$), the presence of GERD increased 3-fold (HR 3.1, 95% CI 1.95–4.95, $p < 0.05$).

In addition, the number of patients with verified bronchiectasis was significantly higher in the main group compared to the control group (6.7% vs. 1.8%). A history of clinically significant bronchiectasis increased the risk of frequent COPD exacerbations by more than 2.5 times (HR 2.59, 95% CI 1.2–5.6, $p < 0.05$). This, in turn, confirms the literature data that in the presence of bronchiectasis, COPD occurs with a greater severity of symptoms, more frequent chronic bronchial infections and exacerbations, as well as a poor prognosis [8].

The risk of community-acquired pneumonia in patients with COPD increases as the severity of the disease increases, while pneumonia itself on the background of COPD is characterized by a more severe course with frequent development of acute respiratory failure [9]. It was found that during the period of COPD exacerbation, community-acquired pneumonia was observed in 1.8% (5) of patients in the control group and in 8.3% (5) of patients in the main group. It was found that the development of pneumonia increased the risk of COPD exacerbation by almost в 1.5 times (HR 1.45, 95% CI 0.771–2.741, $p < 0.05$).

Recommendations given to patients at discharge from the hospital were studied in detail. Despite the fact that smoking remains the main cause of COPD development and progression, and smoking cessation is considered very significant for patients, only 42.8% of patients in the control group and 36.4% of patients in the main group received recommendations for quitting smoking at discharge.

In 74% (199) of cases in the control group, inhaled glucocorticoids (ICS) were prescribed as monotherapy or in combination with bronchodilators on an outpatient бронходилататорамиbasis. CAccording to current clinical guidelines, only 44.7% (89) of such prescriptions could be considered justified. In the main group, IGCS in combination with bronchodilators were prescribed in 77.1% (108) of cases, of which only 49.1% (53) met current clinical recommendations.

Despite the fact that the majority of patients had both hypertension and diabetes mellitus, в 2.6% (7) in the control group and 5% (7) in the main group were recommended to continue taking prednisone at an average dose of 17.86 ± 2.86 mg per day and 19.64 ± 4.64 mg per day on an outpatient basis, respectively, with a gradual reduction in the dose and discontinuation of the drug.

Most patients with severe COPD develop hypoxemia and chronic respiratory failure, which can lead to a decrease in the quality of life, cognitive impairment, and decompensation of the pathology of the cardiovascular system. Long-term oxygen therapy (LTOT) on an outpatient basis using an oxygen concentrator was recommended in 4.5% of patients in the control group and 5% of patients in the main group. Despite this, half of the patients in the control group and 66.7% of the patients in the main group who had indications for LTOT were not recommended to use an oxygen concentrator on an outpatient basis.

To obtain more reliable data on the dynamics of the severity of ventilation disorders, it is necessary to study Spirometry during remission of the disease, but only in 51.2% (87) in the control group and 31.2% (29) in the main group, outpatient spirometry was recommended.

Seasonal influenza vaccination was recommended in 15.7% (42) of cases in the control group and 19.2% (27) of cases in the main group, while pneumococcal vaccination was recommended in only 11.2% (30) and 15.7% (22) of cases, respectively.

Chronic hypoxia in patients with severe COPD may affect adherence to therapy, lead to refusal of physical activity, and changes in the inhalation technique [10]. Non-drug therapy and rehabilitation have the greatest impact on the frequency of exacerbations, but in practice they are not used enough. When analyzing medical records, it was found that only 11.2% (30) of patients in the control group and 9.3% (13) of patients in the main group were given recommendations for maintaining physical activity and respiratory gymnastics.

4. Conclusions

1. Based on the results obtained in the course of the study, it is possible to identify risk factors for repeated hospitalizations in chronic obstructive pulmonary disease: male gender, age over 70 years, smoking duration of 40 years or more, COPD experience of at least 10 years, the presence of three or more concomitant diseases, defects in hospital therapy (inadequate bronchodilator therapy, unjustified treatment), excessive administration of parenteral glucocorticoids and methylxanthines (eufillin), defects in oxygen therapy and antimicrobial treatment regimens, insufficient adherence to treatment at the outpatient stage, including due to inadequate recommendations for treatment at discharge, as well as recommendations for quitting smoking, physical activity and rehabilitation, and lack of proper monitoring of inhalation techniques.

2. The identified risk factors in most cases are considered unmodifiable, so due importance should be given to optimizing treatment and monitoring adherence, as well as non-drug treatment in the form of early smoking cessation, physical and psychological rehabilitation to maintain patients' physical activity.

3. The revealed violations of the quality of medical care provided to patients with severe exacerbations of COPD requiring repeated hospitalizations indicate an insufficient level of knowledge of hospital internists, which requires strengthening the active implementation of the provisions of the federal clinical recommendations on chronic obstructive pulmonary disease in real medical practice.

Funding

The study had no sponsorship.

Conflict of interest

The authors declare no conflict of interest.

Author details

Aigoul Zinnatullina* and Rustem Khamitov
Kazan State Medical University, Kazan, Russian Federation

*Address all correspondence to: aigoul-zinnatullina.rust@mail.ru

References

[1] Lorenz J, Bals R, Dreher M, et al. Exacerbation of COPD. Pneumologie. 2017;**71**(5):269-289. DOI: 10.1055/s-0043-106559

[2] Global Initiative for Chronic Obstructive Lung Disease. Global strategy for the diagnosis, management, and prevention of chronic pulmonary disease; 2021. Available from: https://goldcopd.org/2021-gold-reports/. [Accessed: January 14, 2021]

[3] Chuchalin AG, Belevsky AS, Zhestkov AV et al. Chronic obstructive pulmonary disease: Clinical recommendations. 2018. Available from: https://spulmo.ru/upload/federal_klinicheskie_rekomendaciy_hobl/. [Accessed: January 5, 2021]. (in Russian)

[4] Martynov AI, Malyavin AG, Adasheva TV et al. Diagnosis and treatment of patients with chronic obstructive pulmonary disease and arterial hypertension: National clinical guidelines. 2017. Available from: https://www.rnmot.ru/public/uploads/RNMOT/clinical/2017/ [Accessed: January 10, 2021]. (in Russian)

[5] Pilcher J, Weatherall M, Perrin K, et al. Oxygen therapy in acute exacerbations of chronic obstructive pulmonary disease. Expert Review of Respiratory Medicine. 2015;**9**(3):287-293. DOI: 10.1586/17476348.2015.1016503

[6] Gunen H, Hacievliyagil SS, Yetkin O, et al. The role of nebulized budesonide in the treatment of exacerbations of COPD. The European Respiratory Journal. 2014;**44**(1):272. DOI: 10.1183/0903196.00073506

[7] Toledo-Pons N, Cosio BG. Is there room for theophylline in COPD? Archivos de Bronconeumología. 2017;**53**(10):539-540. DOI: 10.1016/j.arbr.2017.05.019

[8] Martinez-Garcia MA, Miravitlles M. Bronchiectasis in COPD patients: More than a comorbidity? International Journal of Chronic Obstructive Pulmonary Disease. 2017;**12**:1401-1411. DOI: 10.2147/COPD.S132961

[9] Dvoreckij LI. Community-acquired pneumonia in patients with chronic obstructive pulmonary disease. Prakticheskaya Pulmonologiya. 2015;**2**:17-21 (in Russian)

[10] Storgaard LH, Hockey HU, Laursen BS, et al. Long-term effects of oxygen-enriched high-flow nasal cannula treatment in COPD patients with chronic hypoxemic respiratory failure. International Journal of Chronic Obstructive Pulmonary Disease. 2018;**16**(13):1195-1205. DOI: 10.2147/COPD.S159666

Chapter 5

Early Warning Signs and Prodromal Symptoms of AECOPD Patients

Buntarika Chatreewatanakul

Abstract

An acute exacerbation of chronic obstructive pulmonary disease (AECOPD) is a major problem leading to the most cause of death in chronic obstructive pulmonary disease (COPD) patients. Most cases of AECOPD occurred at home and outside the hospital. The COPD patients have the pattern of AECOPD according to their individual experiences. When the patients had AECOPD, also the warning signs and prodromal symptoms were happened differently. However, the characteristics of warning signs and prodromal symptoms could be described in three categories: 1) early signs and symptoms, 2) signs and symptoms that make the patients worse, and 3) time of occurrence. If the patients have been ill with COPD for a period of time until they can learn his/her early warning signs and prodromal symptoms of AECOPD by themselves or/and with their caregivers or/and with healthcare professionals, they will be able to quickly recognize their signs and symptoms when they occur and will be able to manage them as soon as according to their competency individually.

Keywords: early warning signs, prodromal symptoms, an acute exacerbation of chronic obstructive pulmonary disease (AECOPD), chronic obstructive pulmonary disease (COPD), characteristics

1. Introduction

Chronic obstructive pulmonary disease (COPD) is currently a pulmonary problem around the word. It is the third leading cause of death in 2020 [1] and now is one of the top three in 2022 [2]. Most deaths of COPD patients are a cause of worsening of symptoms which it was called acute exacerbation or exacerbation of COPD or AECOPD or COPD flare-up. Exacerbations were cause of respiratory failure that induced the COPD patients to receive life support. Most of AECOPD patients have to receive mechanical ventilator and difficult to wean. It effects to prolong intubation and have low quality of life until those patients die. Moreover, more than 50% of COPD treatment costs were related to exacerbations [3, 4] and they are cause of the slow decline of the disease trajectory that make COPD patients often end of life.

An acute exacerbation can be met in all levels of COPD severity, but it usually occurs in the late stage of it. In 2013, forced expiratory volume in one second (FEV_1) is not suggested for categorizing the severities of COPD. In 2016, the exacerbation was the one criterion that used for categorizing the severities of COPD. Nowadays, only FEV_1 is suggested for categorizing the severities of it [2]. AECOPD first appears in GOLD grade 1 and appears most frequently in grade 4. An exacerbation in COPD patients is an acute state of respiratory symptoms that occurs more than normal day such as dyspnea (shortness of breath), cough, sputum, and makes the patients need additional treatment [5–8]. It is similar to clinical trials, it was defined as "an increasing therapy more than regular day or urgent care is needed the using of antibiotics, systemic corticosteroids, or both in the hospital or/and emergency room" [9]. The severity of AECOPD could be classified into three levels: 1) mild, 2) moderate, and 3) severe. First, the mild level is when the COPD patient has an exacerbation but the treatment not change. Second, the moderated level is when an exacerbation occurs, the medication changes. Finally, AECOPD patient must go to the hospital [9, 10].

Most COPD patients unable to remember their AECOPD events. They do not know the signs and symptoms that happen during they face AECOPD state because they have the pattern of AECOPD according to their individual experiences. It is not similar with other COPD patients. They have to know and recognize it by themselves. It seems like AECOPD experiences are quite unclear. If healthcare professional can help COPD patients able to remember signs and symptoms of AECOPD, they will able to manage it successfully and quickly that it does not affect the bad quality of life.

2. Mechanisms of AECOPD

An acute exacerbation among COPD patients often stimulated by dyspnea (Shortness of breathe) that related with respiratory bacteria or viruses infection (which may coexist), environmental pollutants, or unknown factors. Most of respiratory infection can trigger AECOPD that is pneumonia. During exacerbation happened, there is increased hyperinflation and gas trapping, it resulted to reduced expiratory flow, so effect to dyspnea increased. Airflow limitation and air trapping are the cause of dyspnea and more dyspnea is the one symptom of AECOPD. The pathophysiology of COPD involves an inflammation, fibrosis, and luminal exudates in small airways. It is contributed to gas trapping during expiration and effected to decrease FEV_1 and FEV_1/forced vital capacity (FVC) ratio especially more severe disease. Hyperinflation increases end expiratory lung volume (EELV) and reduces inspiratory capacity (IC) such that functional residual capacity increase, particularly during exercise (dynamic hyperinflation), resulted in mechanical disadvantage (inspiratory muscle dysfunction), neuromechanical uncoupling (increased dyspnea), cardiovascular effects and worsening of gas exchange. Moreover, the increasing of ventilator drive and tachypnea stimulate the worsening of expiratory flow limitation and dynamic hyperinflation each other [5, 6].

3. The perception of early warning signs and prodromal symptoms in AECOPD patients

The perception of early warning signs and prodromal symptoms in AECOPD patients is important to prevent and manage exacerbation among COPD patients. It was according to perception of exacerbation in each COPD patient who aware of exacerbation occurred that means it is different recognition in COPD patients individually. Exacerbation was the event that was showed in 'visible' and 'invisible' symptoms. Visible symptoms were presented in struggles to breathe until cannot breathe and invisible symptoms were presented in really bad, massive anxiety, panic attack, and all things worse liked being trapped in a life-threatening situation that is differently in each person.

4. The characteristics of warning signs and prodromal symptoms of AECOPD

The characteristics of warning signs and prodromal symptoms among AECOPD patients is important to prevent and manage exacerbations. It is different recognition in COPD patients. AECOPD state is the event that was showed in 'visible' and 'invisible' symptoms [11]. Visible symptoms were presented in struggles to breathe until cannot breathe and invisible symptoms were presented in really bad, massive anxiety, panic attack, and all things worse like liked being trapped in a life-threatening situation that is differently in each person.

The specific factors influencing recognition of exacerbations were heterogeneity of exacerbations and habituation to symptoms. They made the patients know the beginning of exacerbation symptoms, included increased fatigue, increased respiratory symptoms (coughing, sputum production, and breathlessness), specific pain and fever [12]. As supported by Chin [13], he stated about exacerbation experiences and the awareness of prodromal symptoms in the days preceding an exacerbation that (1) patients had an unique, individual pattern of exacerbation symptoms that recurred with each exacerbation event, (2) two very distinct types of exacerbation presentations: sudden onset and gradual onset, a change from the participant's typical day-to-day COPD symptom variation, exacerbation occurred from a few hours to 2 weeks, it changes individually, (3) treatment for their exacerbation based on the severity of their symptoms, with participants experiencing sudden, severe dyspnea presenting earliest for treatment, and (4) the severity of symptoms in these individuals precipitated a sense of urgency regarding their situation.

Moreover, COPD Foundation and WebMD reported 17 warning signs and symptoms of AECOPD that COPD patients able to know or recognize how much a COPD flare-up will affect them to make decision in how quickly they can be treated for prevention and treatment of an exacerbation before it becomes too severe, until unable to manage those signs and symptoms. They were consisted of (1) cough more than base line, (2) wheezing more than base line, (3) gurgling or rattle breathing, (4) more dyspnea, (5) more shallow breathing or rapid breathing, (6) produce more mucous than base line, (7) change color in the mucus from clear to green/yellow/tan/bloody, (8) excessive sleepy, (9) confusion, (10) swollen ankles and/or feet, (11) loss of appetite, (12) blue tinge to lips or fingertips, (13) yellow or gray skin, (14) difficult to talk, (15) headaches first thing in the morning, (16) abdominal pain, and (17) chest pain [14]. WebMD [15] stated that there are 9 early warning signs of AECOPD, included (1) noisy breathing, (2) irregular breathing, (3) worsening cough, (4) change color in nails or/and skin, (5) problem sleeping and eating, (6) unable to talk, (7) early-morning headaches, (8) swollen ankles or legs or belly pain, and (9) fever. Moreover, if COPD patients have 4 symptoms; (1) chest pain, (2) blue lips or fingers, (3) confuse or get very easily upset, and (4) dyspnea and unable to talk together, they have to visit the doctor and receive the treatment soon because they can start to become severe suddenly. National Institutes of Health (NIH) [16] divided the warning signs of AECOPD quite differently among COPD Foundation and WebMD reported, it divided the warning signs into two groups, included common early signs and other possible signs. The common early signs consisted of three warning signs; (1) trouble catching patients' breathe, (2) noisy and wheezing sounds, and (3) cough, sometimes has more mucus than normal day or change color in the mucus. The other possible signs consisted of 10 warning signs; (1) unable to take deep breathing, (2) difficult to sleep, (3) morning headache, (4) abdominal pain, (5) anxiety, (6) difficult to talk, (7) swollen ankles or legs, (8) gray or pale skin, (9) blue or purple lips or nail tips, and (10) unable to talk in full sentences.

According to above reporters, awareness of warning signs and prodromal symptoms depended on the perception of each patient who has experienced exacerbation individually. Most warning signs and prodromal symptoms, such as increasing of fatigue, cough, sputum production and breathlessness through hours into 2–7 days [3].

Chatreewatanakul et al. [3] studied about exacerbation experiences among COPD Thai patients. In Thailand, COPD is the fourth most common cause of death and the number of deaths due to COPD is increasing every year. In 2012–2014, there were 1421, 1597, and 1619 COPD-related deaths [17]. The mortality of COPD patients increased from 7.7 deaths per one hundred thousand people in 2013 to 11.4 deaths per one hundred thousand people in 2017. Furthermore, there were 8598 deaths/fiscal year and exacerbation is the most cause of death [18], which is the same cause of death as the world's population that a slow decline of the disease trajectory in COPD, punctuated by dramatic exacerbations that often end in unexpected death or unpredictable death [19]. They found that the characteristics of warning signs and prodromal symptoms could be described in three categories: 1) early signs and symptoms, 2) signs and symptoms that make the patients worse, and 3) time of occurrence.

4.1 Early signs and symptoms

COPD patients recognizes warning signs and prodromal symptoms according to their individual experiences. Early signs and symptoms of AECOPD consisted of two types; 1) frequent early signs and symptoms that are coming before cannot breathe and 2) other early possible signs and symptoms that are coming before cannot breathe.

4.1.1 Frequent early signs and symptoms that are coming before cannot breathe

Most COPD patients have three early signs and symptoms that frequent early occurs before the beginning of AECOPD, included: (1) cough, (2) more dyspnea, and (3) cannot exhale. Cough is the most of signs and symptoms that frequent early occurs before the beginning of AECOPD. More dyspnea and cannot exhale are the second and third respectively.

Since the mechanism of an exacerbation in COPD patients makes cough, more dyspnea, and cannot exhale are related each other. AECOPD is often stimulated by dyspnea which related to respiratory tract infection by bacteria or virus infection, environmental pollution, or unknown factors. During exacerbation state, increasing of hyperinflation and gas trapping, reduce expiratory flow, consequently dyspnea increase [5, 6, 20]. When the participants are ill with respiratory bacteria or viral infection, they will have a cough. This sign will induce dyspnea and result in unable to exhale continuously. Finally, this will induce AECOPD occurring.

4.1.2 Other early possible signs and symptoms that are coming before cannot breathe

COPD patients have early possible signs and symptoms that are coming before cannot breathe different individually. There were twenty-three other early possible signs and symptoms, included: (1) edgy/nervous/moody, (2) difficult breathing, (3) increasing cough, (4) cough with sputum, (5) sticky sputum, (6) a lot of sticky clear white mucus, (7) runny nose, (8) sneeze, (9) stuffy nose, (10) feeling tight like something obstructing in the throat, (11) wheezing, (12) inspiratory wheezing, (13) breathe not all over the stomach, (14) dry cough, (15) tinnitus, (16) hoarse voice, (17) change color in sputum, (18) agitation, (19) sick at heart/heart pain, (20) unsettledness, (21) sweating, (22) frequent cough, and (23) leg pain.

Because COPD patients have different durations of illness and comorbidities, they have early possible signs and symptoms that are coming before cannot breathe differently.

4.2 Signs and symptoms that make the patients worse

There are two categories of signs and symptoms that make the patients worse, included: 1) common signs and symptoms that make the patients worse and 2) signs and symptoms that make the patients decide to go to the hospital.

4.2.1 Common signs and symptoms that make the patients worse

There are four signs and symptoms that make AECOPD patients worse: (1) coughing, (2) wheezing, (3) tightness, and (4) difficulty breathing. Coughing is the sign that most participants have experienced before getting worse but some study said that difficulty breathing is the sign of respiratory system illness which will impact COPD patients' immediate response because it results in airflow limitation and air being trapped which are the cause of increased dyspnea until exacerbation occurs.

4.2.2 Signs and symptoms that make the patients decide to go to the hospital

Seven signs and symptoms make AECOPD patients need to receive the treatment from the doctor at the hospital, included: (1) still dyspnea, (2) cannot exhale, (3) cannot inhale, (4) after receiving bronchodilator therapy, still dyspnea, (5) dyspnea until the body shakes, (6) tinnitus, and (7) when wheezing results in dyspnea. Still dyspnea was the most symptom which the participants decided to go to the hospital to receive treatment from the doctor. It is the symptom that AECOPD patients usually unable to control or manage because they have pulmonary function test (PFT); forced expiratory volume in one second/forced vital capacity (FEV1/FVC) $< 0.70\%$ (confirms the presence of airflow limitation). Thus, they have difficulty to control dyspnea.

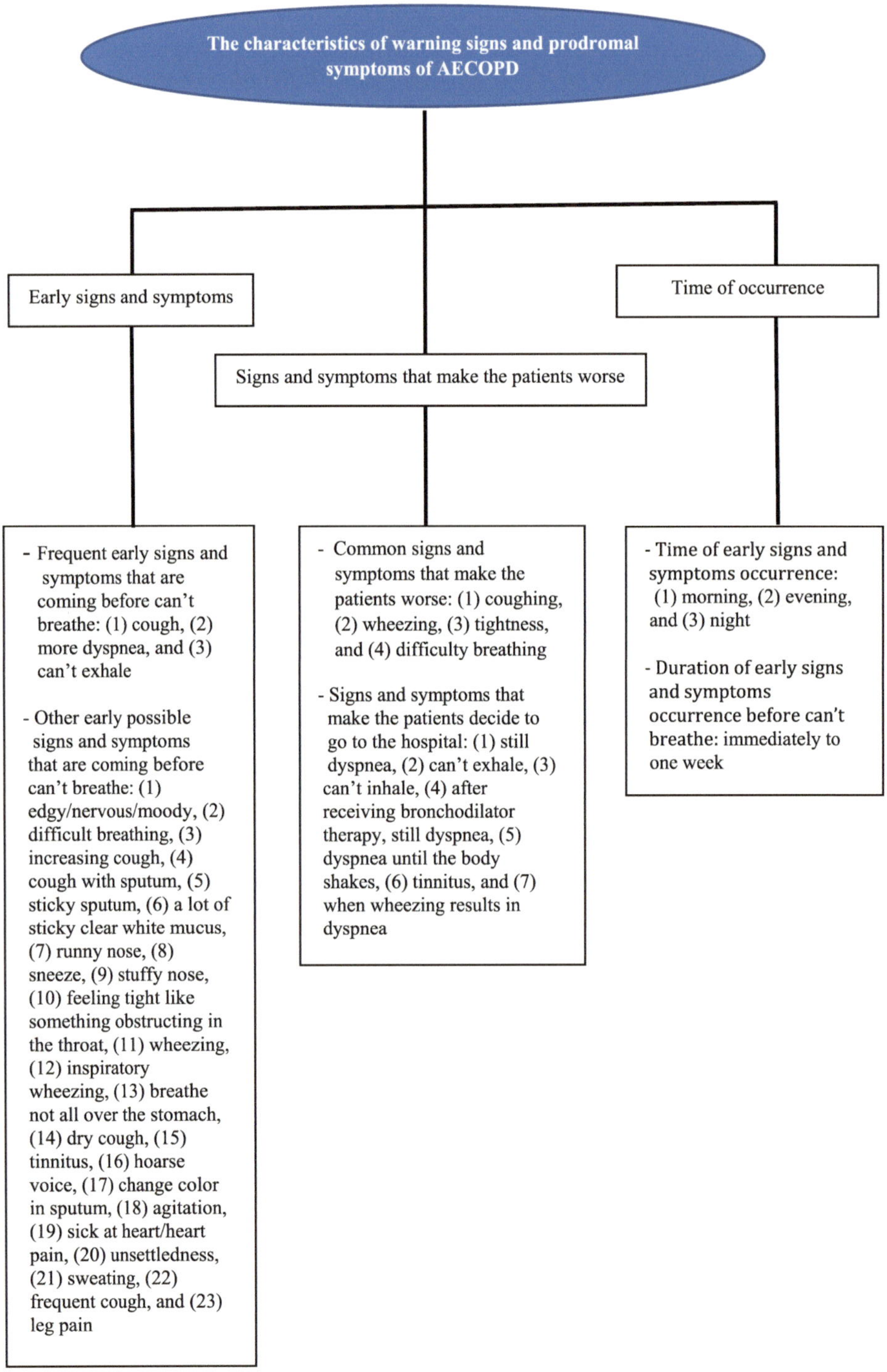

Figure 1.
The characteristics of warning signs and prodromal symptoms of AECOPD.

4.3 Time of occurrence

Time of AECOPD occurrence was included two characteristics: 1) time of early signs and symptoms occurrence and 2) duration of early signs and symptoms occurrence before cannot breathe.

4.3.1 Time of early signs and symptoms occurrence

Most AECOPD patients cannot tell the specific time of early signs and symptoms of exacerbations occurrence. They can be appeared at any time. However, there are some COPD patients who can identify the time of early warning signs and symptoms usually occurring: (1) morning, (2) evening, and (3) night. AECOPD can happen any time. Some patients have signs and symptoms in the morning or/and in the evening or/and in the night or all the day. It occurs different individually.

4.3.2 Duration of early signs and symptoms occurrence before cannot breathe

The duration of early signs and symptoms occurrence before cannot breathe able start from immediately to 1 week. It is different individually that similar to time of early signs and symptoms occurrence.

Although healthcare professionals especially the doctor can know all characteristics of warning signs and prodromal symptoms from COPD patients, they need to assess all signs and symptoms from the patients' caregivers as well. Because some patients cannot tell their all signs and symptoms by themselves. Their caregivers able to help them to inform or encourages the patients to notice those signs and symptoms more clearly. When the clinicians can combine all data from the patients and their caregivers successfully which the data can be gathered early in the onset of exacerbation, it is even better to help the patients manage those signs and symptoms early. As a result, the level of PET dose not decrease rapidly due to each exacerbation which induces the patients to die quickly. The clinicians must also plan for manage those early warning signs and prodromal symptoms early and communicate appropriate methods to manage them with COPD patients and their families by providing the management methods both medication and non-medication treatments or the methods that the patients could learn on their own from previous exacerbation events.

According to early warning signs and prodromal symptoms of AECOPD patients, the characteristics of it can be described in **Figure 1** as follow.

5. Conclusions

In regard to early warning signs and prodromal symptoms of AECOPD patients, COPD patients recognize the warning signs and prodromal symptoms according to their individual experiences. If they able to early recognize the warning signs and prodromal symptoms, they will able to manage it rapidly by themselves or their care givers. As a result, COPD patients will not have the declining of PFT immediately, decreasing of mortality rate, and have a better quality of life. Consequently, healthcare professionals should help and provide the recommendation about early warning signs and prodromal symptoms of AECOPD to COPD patients in order to make it through COPD illness in a period of time during with the patients can learn this knowledge on their own.

6. Recommendations

In healthcare professional area, the various healthcare professionals should help the patients and their care givers by providing the warning signs and prodromal symptoms knowledge appropriately to each COPD patients individually. They should enhance patients care and their management of the early warning signs and prodromal symptoms of AECOPD. Furthermore, supporting AECOPD patients able to plan for recognition of their warning signs and prodromal symptoms by themselves.

Acknowledgements

I express my gratitude to my family members who gave me the moral support. With their love and support, I have been able to achieve my goal. Special thank also Thammasat University, my funding source.

Author details

Buntarika Chatreewatanakul
Faculty of Nursing, Thammasat University, Pathum Thani, Thailand

*Address all correspondence to: buntarika0029@gmail.com

References

[1] Global Initiative for Chronic Obstructive Lung Disease (GOLD). Global Strategy for the Diagnosis, Management, and Prevention of Chronic Obstructive Pulmonary Disease 2020 Report. 2020. Available from: http://www.goldcopd.org/wp-content/uploads/2019/12/GOLD-2020-FINAL-ver1.2-03Dec19_WMV.pdf [Accessed: December 3, 2019]

[2] Global Initiative for Chronic Obstructive Lung Disease (GOLD). Global Strategy for the Diagnosis, Management, and Prevention of Chronic Obstructive Pulmonary Disease 2022 Report. 2022. Available from: https://goldcopd.org/ [Accessed: 14 May, 2022]

[3] Chatreewatanakul B, Othaganont P, Hickman RL. Early symptom recognition and symptom management among exacerbation COPD patients: A qualitative study. Applied Nursing Research. 2022;**63**:151522. DOI: 10.1016/j.apnr.2021.151522

[4] Qureshi H, Sharafkhaneh A, Hanania NA. Chronic obstructive pulmonary disease exacerbations: Latest evidence and clinical implications. Theurapeutic Advances in Chronic Disease. 2014;**5**(5):212-227

[5] Global Initiative for Chronic Obstructive Lung Disease (GOLD). Global Strategy for the Diagnosis, Management, and Prevention of Chronic Obstructive Pulmonary Disease Updated 2016. 2016. Available from: https://www.goldcopd.com [Accessed: August 14, 2016]

[6] Global Initiative for Chronic Obstructive Lung Disease (GOLD). Global Strategy for the Diagnosis, Management, and Prevention of Chronic Obstructive Pulmonary Disease 2017 Report. 2017. Available from: https://www.goldcopd.org/gold-2017-golbal-strategy-diagnosis-management-prevention-copd [Accessed: May 22, 2017]

[7] Global Initiative for Chronic Obstructive Lung Disease (GOLD). Global Strategy for the Diagnosis, Management, and Prevention of Chronic Obstructive Pulmonary Disease 2018 Report. 2018. Available from: https://www.goldcopd.org/gold-2018-golbal-strategy-diagnosis-management-prevention-copd [Accessed: April 28, 2018]

[8] Global Initiative for Chronic Obstructive Lung Disease (GOLD). Global Strategy for the Diagnosis, Management, and Prevention of Chronic Obstructive Pulmonary Disease 2019 Report. 2019. Available from: https://www.goldcopd.org/wp-content/uploads/2018/11/GOLD-2019-v1.6-FINAL-08Nov2018-wms.pdf [Accessed: November 8, 2018]

[9] Criner GJ, Bourbeau J, Diekemper RL, Ouellette DR, Goodridge D, Hernandez P, et al. Prevention of acute exacerbations of COPD. Chest. 2015;**147**(4):894-942

[10] Global Initiative for Chronic Obstructive Lung Disease (GOLD). Global Strategy for the Diagnosis, Management, and Prevention of Chronic Obstructive Pulmonary Disease Updated 2013. 2013. Available from: https://www.goldcopd.com [Accessed: October 7, 2013]

[11] Williams V, Hardinge M, Ryan S, Farmer A. Patients's experience of identifying and managing exacerbations in COPD: A qualitative study. NPJ Primary Care Respiratory Medicine. 2014;**24**:1-6. DOI: 10.1038/npjpcrm.2014.62

[12] Korpershoek YJG, Vervoort SCJM, Nijssen LIT, Trappenburg JCA, Schuurmans MJ. Factors influencing exacerbation-related self-management in patients with COPD: A qualitative study. International Journal of COPD. 2016;**11**:2977-2990

[13] Chin ED. The COPD exacerbation experience: A qualitative descriptive study. Applied Nursing Research. 2017;**38**:38-44

[14] Henderson W. 17 Warning Signs of COPD Exacerbations. 2017. Available from: https://www.copdnewstoday.com [Accessed: 7 October, 2020]

[15] WebMD. Signs of a COPD Flare-Up. 2019. Available from: https://www.webmd.com/ling/10-signs-copd-exacerbation#1 [Accessed: October 7, 2020]

[16] National Institute of Health. COPD flare-ups. 2019. Available from: https://www.medlineplus.gov/ency/patientinstructions/000698.htm [Accessed: October 7, 2020]

[17] Bureau of Non-Communicable Disease, Ministry of Public Health. Annual report 2015. 2015. Available from: https://www.thailand.com/document/file/download/paper-manual/Annual-report-2015.pdf (In Thai) [Accessed: January 5, 2021]

[18] Bureau of Non-Communicable Disease, Ministry of Public Health. Reported mortality of COPD patients on 20th April 2018. 2018. Available from: https://www.hdcservice.moph.go.th/hdc/reports/report.php?source=formated/ncd.php&cat_id=6a1fdf282fd28180eed7d1cfe0155 (In Thai) [Accessed: January 5, 2021]

[19] Spathis A, Booth S. End of life care in chronic obstructive pulmonary disease: in search of a good death. International Journal of COPD. 2008;**3**(1):11-29

[20] O'Donnell DE, Parker CM. COPD exacerbations 3: Phathophysiology. Thorax. 2006;**61**:354-361

Chapter 6

Current and Contemporary Developments in Pulmonary Rehabilitation

Biruk Getahun and Abebe Ayalew Bekel

Abstract

Chronic obstructive pulmonary disease (COPD) is now recognized as a global health problem. It is most usually caused by smoking cigarettes, although it can also be caused by a variety of environmental toxins, noxious gases, fumes, and dust. Pulmonary rehabilitation (PR) is an effective intervention for patients with chronic obstructive pulmonary disease and is recommended by clinical guidelines. It is an important part of the treatment of chronic obstructive pulmonary disease and other chronic respiratory disorders. Pulmonary rehabilitation is a recent approach in respiratory medicine that is defined as an "individually customized and designed, interdisciplinary program of care" for patients with persistent respiratory failure. Patient selection and assessment, psychological support, self-management education, nutritional support, and exercise training (including inspiratory muscle training (IMT) are all important components of pulmonary rehabilitation.

Keywords: pulmonary rehabilitation, respiratory medicine, intervention, chronic respiratory disorder

1. Introduction

Chronic obstructive pulmonary disease (COPD) is characterized by significant functional limitation and high mortality. COPD exacerbations are associated with disease progression and are one of the leading causes of hospitalization and death, emphasizing the necessity of interventions to prevent or mitigate exacerbations. Medication management, patient education, exacerbation action plans, and pulmonary rehabilitation are all important aspects of COPD treatment [1]. Pulmonary rehabilitation, which consists of exercise and self-management education, is considered critical in the treatment of COPD patients. However, these improvements are not maintained long term. At 12 months following pulmonary rehabilitation, measures of exercise capacity, symptoms, and health-related quality of life (HRQoL) have returned toward their pre-rehabilitation values [2]. It is possible that exacerbations in the post-pulmonary rehabilitation period contribute to the lack of sustained benefit at 12 months, but this has not been systematically evaluated. Understanding the effects of exacerbations on long-term results and who is at risk for exacerbations can help with the development of more effective maintenance strategies following pulmonary rehabilitation [1, 2].

2. Definition of pulmonary rehabilitation

Pulmonary rehabilitation (PR), which is a cornerstone in the non-pharmacological management of COPD, is defined by the American Thoracic Society/European Respiratory Society (ATS/ERS) as a "comprehensive intervention based on a thorough patient assessment followed by patient-tailored therapies that include, but are not limited to, exercise training, education, and behavior change, designed to improve the physical and psychological condition of people with chronic respiratory disease [2, 3]. PR is an evidence-based, multidisciplinary, and comprehensive intervention for patients with chronic lung disorders who are symptomatic and have some disability. Through stabilizing or reversing systemic signs of the disease, pulmonary rehabilitation aims to reduce symptoms, optimize functional state, increase participation, and reduce healthcare costs. To put it another way, depending on the stage of the disease, a symptomatic COPD patient has some functional compromise that can be rectified by rehabilitation [3]. In recent years, there has been increasing interest in the role of PR in the acute setting (either during or shortly after a hospital admission for AECOPD) [2].

Health behavior change is vital for optimization and maintenance of benefits from any intervention in chronic care, and PR has taken a lead in implementing strategies

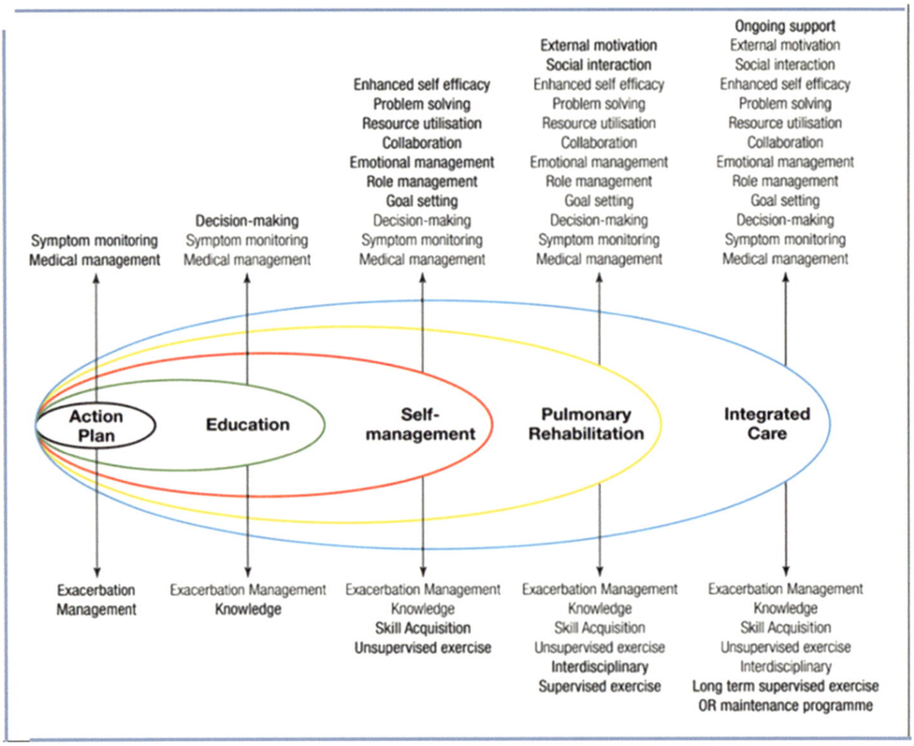

Figure 1.
Spectrum of support for chronic obstructive pulmonary disease [5].

to achieve this goal. This model may provide more clarity on the material and methods used to achieve various levels of support. It aids in the defining of terminology and may assist practitioners in determining a person's requirements and the amount of care necessary [4]. Healthcare professionals interested in the field might use this tool to help construct interventions, identify appropriate outcome measures, and define the intervention in a standardized way. The most comprehensive PR program, which includes self-management, should be prioritized for the most severe patients, which is referred to as integrated care (**Figure 1**). The minimal "action plan" intervention may be sufficient for less complicated patients with basic demands [5]. Long-term health maintenance in the face of a progressive disease is challenging. Several studies have suggested that the only approach to maintain changes in health status is to change one's behavior. Cognitive behavioral approaches have been offered as therapies that could help people change their habits. The text recognizes self-efficacy as a critical component of behavior change. Behavior modification may be more successful if weaknesses in self-efficacy are identified and manipulated [5].

3. Rationale and outcomes

Recent evidence-based reviews have confirmed the effect of PR on COPD outcomes, including improved exercise capacity, reduced dyspnea and leg discomfort, improved quality of life (QoL), enhanced self-efficacy, and improved activities of daily living. PR has positive impacts on lung health without having any discernible impact on standard lung function tests like forced expiratory volume in one second (FEV1) [3]. The fact that PR lessens the systemic symptoms of COPD and its prevalent comorbidities provides a clear explanation for this discrepancy. Peripheral muscle dysfunction as a result of physical inactivity or systemic inflammation, muscle wasting, inadequate self-management skills, anxiety, and depression are all significant systemic effects of COPD [5]. Systemic effects and comorbid conditions contribute to the disease burden and might be amenable to therapy. For example, physical conditioning of leg muscles through exercise training reduces lactate production and decreases ventilator load. COPD patients with a decreased ventilatory load can breathe more slowly during exercise, reducing dynamic hyperinflation. These effects usually reduce exertional dyspnea, even without a change in FEV1 [3, 5].

4. Essential components of pulmonary rehabilitation A

Patient selection and assessment, psychological support, self-management education, nutritional support, and exercise training (including inspiratory muscle training (IMT) are all important components of PR (**Figure 2**) [5]. One of the actual PR program is a multidisciplinary home-based program. In this program, breathing retraining consists of pursed-lip breathing and diaphragmatic breathing performed in the supine or sitting positions. Exercise training includes upper- and lower-extremity exercise, respiratory muscle stretching calisthenics, level walking, and IMT. Patients with COPD participate in educational activities such as lectures on respiratory conditions, dyspnea control, medication, equipment use, diet, stress management, relaxation techniques, at-home exercise, and the idea and advantages of PR [3, 6]. Each patient receives periodic home visits from a registered nurse practitioner who informs them about the function of PR. This PR program is different from recent home-based

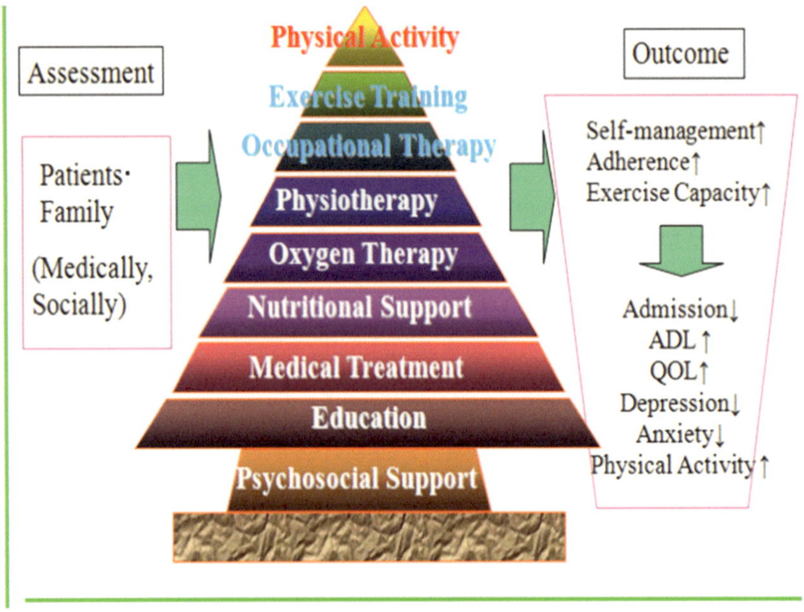

Figure 2.
Basic construction of pulmonary rehabilitation [5].

PR programs in the point of low-intensity exercise program including such as respiratory muscle stretching calisthenics and low-intensity IMT [5–7].

4.1 Self-management education

Education in self-management is a crucial and essential component of PR. It stimulates active engagement in healthcare and supports self-efficacy. It has been demonstrated that self-management education is very helpful in enhancing health and lowering healthcare utilization. It is typically given in a one-on-one or small group environment [8]. Individual educational needs are identified during an initial assessment and reviewed throughout the PR program [5, 8]. Key parts of self-management education include discussions of advance directives and counseling on the early identification and treatment of COPD exacerbations [9].

4.2 Psychosocial support

The burden of advanced respiratory disease is exacerbated by anxiety, sadness, coping issues, and a lack of self-efficacy. Despite the lack of evidence to support psychosocial therapies as a single therapeutic modality in COPD patients, complete PR programs that include these types of interventions reap advantages [10].

Comprehensive PR leads to small- to moderate-scale improvements in anxiety and dyspnea when compared to usual therapy, according to research. PR programs differ in their use of psychosocial and behavioral interventions, but they frequently contain educational sessions or support groups that concentrate on coping mechanisms and stress management. These support groups also promote participation from patients' loved ones and friends. Patients with severe mental illness should be referred for the proper treatment [5, 11].

4.3 Exercise training

4.3.1 Exercise training for upper and lower extremities

A crucial component of PR programs is exercise training. Exercise training has been demonstrated to be the most effective method for improving muscle strength. It is also likely to increase motivation for exercise, reduce mood disorders, reduce symptoms, and improve cardiovascular health. Endurance and resistance training should be a part of PR programs, according to recent major guidelines, which are the essential components of exercise training programs for COPD patients. Although none of the recommendations give clear, accurate, and precise recommendations for full exercise training, they all support endurance training at least three to five times per week at a rate more than 60% of one's maximum heart rate. Although it is advised to exercise for at least 20 minutes and for a target program duration of up to 12 weeks, there is disagreement on initial workloads, increasing the exercise load, or program duration [5, 11].

PR requires a comprehensive workout program that includes upper- and lower-extremity endurance training as well as strength training. COPD is a disease of the peripheral muscles, characterized by a loss of mass, changes in fiber-type distribution, and a reduction in metabolic capacity, all of which contribute to exercise intolerance. Exercise training may be able to help with these issues. Higher degrees of exercise training are linked to a stronger physiologic training impact, dose-dependent changes in oxidative enzymes in limb muscles, and increased exercise capacity [11].

Exercise training is based on the main concepts of intensity (higher intensity produces better results), specificity (only the muscles that have been trained show an effect), and reversibility (only the muscles that have been trained show an effect) (cessation of regular exercise training results in a decrease in training effect) [6]. Although patients with COPD often have ventilatory limitations to maximal exercise, high training targets can nevertheless have a physiologic training impact. Exercise intensity of 60 to 80% of the patient's peak work rate is often feasible [5].

Another crucial aspect of exercise training is strength training, which also offers potential advantages. Strength training can be helpful for patients who cannot withstand intense exercise regimens. Some patients might be able to train at higher intensities by maximizing bronchodilation, doing interval training (i.e. switching between high and low intensities), and taking oxygen supplements [4, 5]. The optimal training duration has not been determined; rather, it is based on how each patient is doing. A successful PR program should continue at least 8 weeks (with three to four sessions each week), following the GOLD (Global Initiative for Chronic Obstructive Lung Disease) criteria, but the longer the better [12].

Although, high-intensity exercise training is effective and ideal, the rate of implementation and continuation is low especially in home-based PR setting. Therefore, low-intensity exercise training is a realistic choice in home-based PR setting [5].

4.3.2 Inspiratory muscle training (IMT)

COPD patients have respiratory muscle weakness, which contributes to hypercapnia, dyspnea, nocturnal oxygen desaturation, and reduced walking distance. Diaphragm work is increased in COPD patients during exercise, and COPD patients use a greater proportion of the maximum inspiratory pressure (PI max) than healthy subjects [5]. This pattern of breathing is closely related to the dyspnea sensation during exercise and might potentially induce respiratory muscle fatigue [13].

Respiratory muscle training is a part of rehabilitation in selected patients with COPD. Respiratory strength has been found to correlate with improved pulmonary function, reduction of dyspnea severity, improved exercise tolerance, and enhanced functionality and quality of life [9]. By boosting type II fibers, which leads to a decrease in inspiratory time and an increase in expiratory time, inspiratory muscle training (IMT) is thought to help the diaphragm contract. Since hyperinflation is anticipated to eventually decrease, IMT is believed to have an effect on dyspnea without significantly changing inspiratory pressure [13, 14].

4.3.3 New advances in the exercise training

There have been numerous new developments in exercise training in recent years, which is a crucial part of PR. In patients with COPD and physical comorbidities, water-based exercise training has been demonstrated to be noticeably more successful than land-based exercise training and control in raising peak and endurance exercise capacity and improving health-related quality of life (HRQoL) [4, 5]. Compared to level walking, downhill walking causes higher quadriceps low-frequency fatigue in COPD patients, who also experience reduced cardio-respiratory expenses [15]. It has been proposed that downhill walking can be a beneficial component of a thorough rehabilitation program [16]. It has also been demonstrated that eccentric exercise therapy, such as downhill walking, improves bodily functions and HRQoL and increases the size of the thigh muscles. Whole-body vibration has been proven to be a useful tool for strengthening muscles and as a potential means of reducing wasting and weakening. Patients with COPD who are bedridden and unable to receive physical physiotherapy might gain anything. The use of whole-body vibration proved safe and practical, and the method results in more energy use [5, 14].

4.4 Nutritional support

Patients with COPD who are underweight have worse lung health, less diaphragmatic mass, less exercise tolerance, and a greater mortality rate than those who are properly fed. Nutritional supplementation could be beneficial for their comprehensive care [6] to evaluate how dietary supplementation affects anthropometric measurements, lung function, strength, endurance, functional exercise capacity, and HRQoL in COPD. If a benefit is seen, subgroup analysis should be done to determine the treatment plans and subpopulations that show the most promise [5].

5. Physical activity in COPD

Using indirect calorimetry techniques like doubly labeled water or metabolic carts, daily physical activity can be reported as an overall metric of active energy expenditure. The duration, frequency, and intensity of physical activity are not quantified by the doubly labeled water approach, despite the fact that it is considered a criteria method [6, 17]. Metabolic cart systems that measure expired O_2 and CO_2 are, however, not suitable for long-term usage. Physical activity monitors can also be used to directly track physical activity [2].

In general, pedometers, accelerometers, and integrated multi-sensor systems are the three classes of activity monitors that are being utilized more frequently in populations with chronic diseases (like COPD). Pedometers are gadgets that solely measure in the vertical plane mechanically or digitally to quantify the number of steps taken [5]. This is only a small amount of exercise. One, two, or three directions of acceleration can be detected using accelerometers (uni-, bi-, or triaxial accelerometers). These tools enable measurement of movement quality, amount, and intensity [5, 15]. In an effort to improve physical activity assessments, integrated multisensory systems combine accelerometry with various sensors that record physiological reactions to exercise (such as heart rate or skin temperature). Technology has advanced to the point that a variety of activity monitors are now readily available to measure physical activity [18].

Physical activity in patients with COPD is dependent on many factors, including physiological, behavioral, social, environmental, and cultural factors. Only a weak association exists between daily physical activity and post-bronchodilator FEV1. Dynamic hyperinflation, which highly correlates with exertional dyspnea in COPD, and daily physical activity, however, have a strong inverse relationship [19]. Performance on lower-limb muscle function tests and field exercise tests correlates better with physical activity in COPD than resting lung function testing does. Lower levels of physical activity are related to daily COPD symptoms (such as dyspnea and fatigue). In patients with COPD, the relationship between impaired health status and physical activity is minimal to moderate. Interestingly, this link between a drop in physical activity and a decline in health status in COPD patients was validated in a 5-year longitudinal observational study [3, 5, 13].

Levels of physical exercise influence critical outcomes in COPD. Hospitalization due to an exacerbation is connected with lower levels of physical activity. 59 After adjusting for age, FEV1, and prior hospitalizations, a drop in physical activity over time also predicts COPD-related hospitalization in addition to baseline levels of physical activity [20]. Even after accounting for or taking into consideration pertinent confounding factors, people with COPD who engage in less physical activity have a higher chance of dying from any cause. Mortality is also predicted by a decline in physical activity over time. Physical activity has been incorporated as a factor in multidimensional predictive scores for all-cause and respiratory mortality, exacerbations, and COPD-related hospitalization in stable COPD patients, reflecting these substantial relationships [18, 21]. The importance of encouraging physical activity in the early stages of COPD, with a target of more than 2 hours per week, is highlighted by these outcome studies [5, 18].

5.1 The effects of pulmonary rehabilitation on physical activity in COPD

Exercise training and education, which work to transform behavior by encouraging self-efficacy, are the cornerstones of PR. The increases in exercise capacity shown in the rehabilitation facility would ideally translate into increases in physical activity in the home and community settings for PR to have its best long-term impact [19, 22]. To obtain a large and long-lasting increase in daily physical activity in COPD patients, both improvements in exercise capacity and adaptive behavioral modifications are required. The definition of physical activity (which is a distinct component from exercise capacity), its prevalence in COPD, its objective assessment, risk factors for physical inactivity, and potential methods to maintain or develop the physical strength components are all included in this clinical review. In stable COPD patients, PR has likely the biggest favorable impact on exercise capacity of any contemporary medication [22].

An interdisciplinary strategy including pulmonary medicine, rehabilitation sciences, social sciences, and behavioral sciences is required to alter physical activity behavior in COPD patients. The data in this succinct clinical review show that people with COPD are typically quite sedentary, and that this lack of physical exercise is bad for both the quality and quantity of life [23, 24]. Therefore, a major objective of PR must be to make increasing efforts to better understand the factors that influence physical activity as well as practical ways to enhance this characteristic. The ATS/ERS Official Statement on PR now lists physical activity as one of the primary outcome metrics of PR programs [25].

6. Neuromuscular electrical stimulation (NMES)

Neuromuscular electrical stimulation (NMES) is one of the more recent forms of rehabilitation that works by depolarizing motor neurons to apply an electric current through electrodes implanted on the skin over the targeted muscles, passively stimulating the contraction of the peripheral muscles [26]. It aims to elicit favorable training effects in patients who are unable to take part in PR programs without inducing dyspnea. The stimulation frequency ranges from 8 to 120 Hz, and the stimulation pulse lasts typically between 250 and 400 s. The intensity is steadily increased throughout the entire stimulation, ranging from 10 to 100 mA, depending on the patient's personal tolerance. NMES increased quadriceps strength and exercise capacity, according to a meta-analysis published in 2016. However, there was no statistically significant change in the degree of health-related quality of life in patients with moderate-to-severe COPD [14, 27, 28]. NMES has been linked to a reduction in muscle oxidative stress and an increase in type II fiber cross-sectional area with a decrease in type I fiber cross-sectional area in a number of investigations on COPD patients [29]. NMES could be used during times of exacerbation and during admission to the ICU for acute COPD exacerbation because it has a low influence on ventilation, heart rate, and dyspnea [14].

7. Noninvasive mechanical ventilation (NIMV)

Exercise tolerance is increased by noninvasive mechanical ventilation (NIMV), because the acute stress on the respiratory muscles is lessened. These mechanisms explain why the impact of NIMV on PR results has been studied in various studies where NIMV was used at night or during exercise training [30]. The effect of NIMV during exercise training as part of PR was examined in a review of the Cochrane Database, and it was found that doing so increased lower limb exercise capacity and permitted exercise at higher training intensities [31, 32]. No studies looked into the impact of NIMV during exercise training on physical activity, and there was no conclusive evidence regarding quality of life. It has also been demonstrated that nocturnal NIMV following PR increased exercise tolerance and quality of life in patients with severe COPD, presumably by giving the respiratory muscles a rest at night. The ERS/ATS guidelines state that NIMV may be used as an additional therapy to unload the respiratory muscles so that certain patients with severe chronic respiratory disease who do not respond well to exercise can intensify their exercise regimen [14, 30].

8. Conclusion

Pulmonary rehabilitation, a non-pharmacologic therapy, has become the standard of care for COPD patients. It is a comprehensive, multidisciplinary, patient-centered intervention that includes patient assessment, exercise training, self-management education, and psychosocial support. Positive outcomes from pulmonary rehabilitation include increased exercise tolerance, reduced dyspnea and anxiety, increased self-efficacy, and improvement in health-related quality of life. An interdisciplinary approach including pulmonary medicine, rehabilitation sciences, social sciences, and behavioral sciences is required to alter physical activity behavior in COPD patients. Primary care physicians, nurse practitioners, and all other allied healthcare providers require greater education and learning opportunities about the procedure and advantages of pulmonary rehabilitation. Future research will also need to address the viability and security of pulmonary rehabilitation. Increasing the number of healthcare professionals, patients' understanding of and access to pulmonary rehabilitation, and improving the program's quality are key processes essential to attaining these goals.

Conflict of interest

The authors declare that they have no competing interest.

Author details

Biruk Getahun[1]* and Abebe Ayalew Bekel[2]

1 Department of Medical Physiology, School of Medicine, College of Medicine and Health Sciences, Bahir Dar University, Bahir Dar, Ethiopia

2 Department of Human Anatomy, School of Medicine, College of Medicine and Health Sciences, Bahir Dar University, Bahir Dar, Ethiopia

*Address all correspondence to: birukkgetahun@gmail.com

References

[1] Wageck B, Cox NS, McDonald CF, Burge AT, Mahal A, Hill CJ, et al. The impact of COPD exacerbations in the year following pulmonary rehabilitation: Secondary analysis of a randomised controlled trial. International Journal of Chronic Obstructive Pulmonary Disease. 2020;**15**:3423

[2] Jones SE, Barker RE, Nolan CM, Patel S, Maddocks M, Man WD. Pulmonary rehabilitation in patients with an acute exacerbation of chronic obstructive pulmonary disease. Journal of Thoracic Disease. 2018;**10**(Suppl 12):S1390

[3] Sharma BB, Singh V. Pulmonary rehabilitation: An overview. Lung India: Official Organ of Indian Chest Society. 2011;**28**(4):276

[4] Seymour JM, Moore L, Jolley CJ, Ward K, Creasey J, Steier JS, et al. Outpatient pulmonary rehabilitation following acute exacerbations of COPD. Thorax. 2010;**65**(5):423-428

[5] Shioya T, Iwakura M, Kawagoshi A. Recent advances in pulmonary rehabilitation for patients with COPD. Pulmonary Research and Respiratory Medicine. 2017:S7-S19

[6] Troosters T, Blondeel A, Janssens W, Demeyer H. The past, present and future of pulmonary rehabilitation. Respirology. 2019;**9**:830-837

[7] Singh S, Bolton C, Nolan C. BTS Guidance for Pulmonary Rehabilitation–Reopening Services for the 'Business as Usual 'Participants. 2020. Available from: www. brit-thoracic. org. uk/about-us/covid-19-resumption-and-continuation-of-respiratory-services

[8] Selzler AM, Simmonds L, Rodgers WM, Wong EY, Stickland MK. Pulmonary rehabilitation in chronic obstructive pulmonary disease: Predictors of program completion and success. COPD: Journal of Chronic Obstructive Pulmonary Disease. 2012;**9**(5):538-545

[9] Alfarroba S, Rodrigues F, Papoila AL, Santos AF, Morais L. Pulmonary rehabilitation in COPD according to global initiative for chronic obstructive lung disease categories. Respiratory Care. 2016;**61**(10): 1331-1340

[10] Porszasz J, Brusasco V. Current status of pulmonary rehabilitation: Introductory remarks on pulmonary rehabilitation, the importance and the practice. COPD: Journal of Chronic Obstructive Pulmonary Disease. 2018;**15**(3):215-218

[11] Puhan MA, Gimeno-Santos E, Cates CJ, Troosters T. Pulmonary rehabilitation following exacerbations of chronic obstructive pulmonary disease. Cochrane Database of Systematic Reviews. 2016;**12**

[12] Holland AE, Cox NS, Houchen-Wolloff L, Rochester CL, Garvey C, ZuWallack R, et al. Defining modern pulmonary rehabilitation. An Official American Thoracic. 2018;**18**(5):e12-e29

[13] Wouters EF, Posthuma R, Koopman M, Liu WY, Sillen MJ, Hajian B, et al. An update on pulmonary rehabilitation techniques for patients with chronic obstructive pulmonary disease. Expert Review of Respiratory Medicine. 2020;**14**(2):149-161

[14] Candemir I. Advances in pulmonary rehabilitation for chronic obstructive

pulmonary disease and associated conditions. COPD–an update in pathogenesis and clinical management. Intech. 2018;**21**:131-151

[15] Puhan MA, Spaar A, Frey M, Turk A, Brändli O, Ritscher D, et al. Early versus late pulmonary rehabilitation in chronic obstructive pulmonary disease patients with acute exacerbations: A randomized trial. Respiration. 2012;**83**(6):499-506

[16] Santus P, Bassi L, Radovanovic D, Airoldi A, Raccanelli R, Triscari F, et al. Pulmonary rehabilitation in COPD: A reappraisal (2008-2012). Pulmonary Medicine. 2013;**9**:2013

[17] McCarthy B, Casey D, Devane D, Murphy K, Murphy E, Lacasse Y. Pulmonary rehabilitation for chronic obstructive pulmonary disease. Cochrane Database of Systematic Reviews. 2015;**2**

[18] Young P, Dewse M, Fergusson W, Kolbe J. Respiratory rehabilitation in chronic obstructive pulmonary disease: Predictors of nonadherence. The European Respiratory Journal. 1999;**13**(4):855-859

[19] Snyder N, Wilson R, Finch L, Gallant B, Landa C, Frankel D, et al. The role of occupational therapy in pulmonary rehabilitation programs: Protocol for a scoping review. JMIR Research Protocols. 2021;**10**(7):e30244

[20] Kjærgaard JL, Juhl CB, Lange P, Wilcke JT. Early pulmonary rehabilitation after acute exacerbation of COPD: A randomised controlled trial. ERJ Open Research. 2020;**6**:1

[21] Troosters T, Gosselink R, Janssens W, Decramer MJ. Exercise training and pulmonary rehabilitation: New insights and remaining challenges. European Respiratory Review. 2010;**19**(115):24-29

[22] Egan C, Deering BM, Blake C, Fullen BM, McCormack NM, Spruit MA, et al. Short term and long term effects of pulmonary rehabilitation on physical activity in COPD. Respiratory Medicine. 2012;**106**(12):1671-1679

[23] Sciriha A, Montefort S. Pulmonary rehabilitation: Insight into current trends. Malta Medical Journal. 2010

[24] Spruit MA, Pitta F, McAuley E, ZuWallack RL, Nici L. Pulmonary rehabilitation and physical activity in patients with chronic obstructive pulmonary disease. American Journal of Respiratory and Critical Care Medicine. 2015;**192**(8):924-933

[25] Rochester CL, Vogiatzis I, Holland AE, Lareau SC, Marciniuk DD, Puhan MA, et al. Enhancing implementation, use, and delivery of pulmonary. An Official American Thoracic Society/European Respiratory Society. 2015;**192**(11):1373-1386

[26] Mekki M, Paillard T, Sahli S, Tabka Z, Trabelsi Y. Effect of adding neuromuscular electrical stimulation training to pulmonary rehabilitation in patients with chronic obstructive pulmonary disease: Randomized clinical trial. Clinical Rehabilitation. 2019;**33**(2):195-206

[27] Neder JA, Sword D, Ward SA, Mackay E, Cochrane LM, Clark CJ. Home based neuromuscular electrical stimulation as a new rehabilitative strategy for severely disabled patients with chronic obstructive pulmonary disease (COPD). Thorax. 2002;**57**(4):333-337

[28] Giavedoni S, Deans A, McCaughey P, Drost E, MacNee W, Rabinovich RA. Neuromuscular electrical stimulation prevents muscle function deterioration in exacerbated COPD:

A pilot study. Respiratory Medicine. 2012;**106**(10):1429-1434

[29] Gloeckl R, Schneeberger T, Jarosch I, Kenn K. Pulmonary rehabilitation and exercise training in chronic obstructive pulmonary disease. Deutsches Ärzteblatt International. 2018;**115**(8):117

[30] Cui L, Liu H, Sun L. Multidisciplinary respiratory rehabilitation in combination with non-invasive positive pressure ventilation in the treatment of elderly patients with severe chronic obstructive pulmonary disease. Pakistan Journal of Medical Sciences. 2019;**35**(2):500

[31] Köhnlein T, Schönheit-Kenn U, Winterkamp S, Welte T, Kenn K. Noninvasive ventilation in pulmonary rehabilitation of COPD patients. Respiratory Medicine. 2009;**103**(9): 1329-1336

[32] Barakat S, Michele G, Nesme P, Nicole V, Guy A. Effect of a noninvasive ventilatory support during exercise of a program in pulmonary rehabilitation in patients with COPD. International Journal of Chronic Obstructive Pulmonary Disease. 2007;**2**(4):585

Chapter 7

New Perspectives in Pharmacological Therapy for COPD: Phenotype Classification and Corticosteroids with Bronchodilators

Hiroaki Kume, Ryuki Yamada and Yuki Sato

Abstract

Chronic obstructive lung disease (COPD) is heterogeneous and complex. Symptoms and pathophysiological disorders overlap between COPD and asthma. To progress the management of COPD, patients with COPD should be classified by distinct clinical phenotypes. These groupings derived from multiple dimensions including clinical, physiologic, imaging, and endotyping determine clusters of patients with common characteristics that relate to clinically meaningful outcomes such as symptoms, exacerbations, response to therapy, and disease progression (stratified medicine). Moreover, since several phenotypes can coexist in individual patients with COPD, an approach due to therapeutic target identified phenotypes and endotypes (treatable traits) has been proposed as an advanced therapy recently (precision medicine). Airway eosinophilia and airway hyperresponsiveness, which are hallmarks of asthma, are developed in some patients with COPD, independent of asthma. It is perhaps meaningful to classify COPD according to airway eosinophilia and airway hyperresponsiveness as phenotypes and to put these phenotypes into focus as treatable traits. These phenotypes are closely related to frequency of exacerbations and reactivity to inhaled corticosteroids with bronchodilators in therapy for COPD. Hence, research for phenotype classification can play a fundamental role for development of the management and treatment for COPD.

Keywords: COPD, phenotypes, treatable traits, airway eosinophilic inflammation, airway hyperresponsiveness

1. Introduction

Chronic obstructive lung disease (COPD) is defined as a common, preventable, and treatable disease that is characterized by persistent respiratory symptoms (shortness of breath, chronic cough, sputum production) and by airway obstruction (airflow limitation) that will not return to the normal range [1]. It is considered that COPD is complex and heterogeneous in symptoms, disease progression, functional outcomes, and response to therapies based on the etiology, pathogenesis, and type of lung pathology [2]. To address this complexity and heterogeneity, it is desirable to meaningfully identify and classify groups of patients with similar clinical characteristics, prognosis, and/or therapeutic needs, referred to as clinical phenotypes. However, it has not established to classify patients with COPD into defined subtypes according to distinct phenotypes. The Genetic Epidemiology of Chronic Obstructive Pulmonary Disease (COPDGene) study, which is a longitudinal cohort study of more than 10,000 smokers, is being carried out to identify the etiology, progression, and heterogeneity of COPD. This cohort study is probably useful for research and development of treatable trait toward precision medicine or personalized medicine for COPD [3–5].

Chronic lung inflammation, which is caused by cigarette smoke and other environmental exposures (biomass fuel, air pollution etc.), contributes to the pathogenesis of this disease. This chronic lung inflammation related to neutrophils and macrophages is normal response in many people, but appears to be modified in patients who develop COPD, leading to emphysema and small airway fibrosis, which are essential characteristics in pathology of this disease. COPD is diagnosed only by persistent airflow limitation in spirometry, but other variables in lung function test may be relevant to diagnosis and prognosis of this disease. Since not only FEV_1 but also FEV_1/FVC physiologically decreases with age, the fixed cutoff point for FEV_1/FVC ratio may be inaccurate to use for diagnosis of COPD. Airflow limitation is progressive, and a decline of FEV_1 varies in each patient.

The pathological alterations cause not only airflow limitation mediated by the loss of alveolar attachment to the small airways but also gas trapping (an increase in residual volume (RV) or a decrease in inspiratory capacity (IC)). Moreover, these structural alterations also cause a decrease in lung elastic recoil (a reduction in dynamic elastance). Since COPD is associated with not only small airway but also alveolar disease [6], some patients with COPD have a low diffusing capacity of the lung for carbon monoxide (DL_{CO}). It has been recognized that chronic airflow obstruction could be seen in a variety of overlapping conditions among airway diseases, most notably in patients with COPD and asthma [7, 8]. The overlap of asthma and COPD has been proposed as a distinct COPD phenotype, refers to a set of observable characteristics of an organism.

When infections or heart failure occurs in patients, the stable periods of COPD may be interrupted by acute worsening of respiratory symptoms (exacerbations). Moreover, significant chronic diseases are concomitant with most patients with COPD (comorbidity) [9]. The prognosis of each patient with COPD is probably dependent on frequency of exacerbations and coexisting diseases. Hence, COPD is a heterogeneous disease in symptoms, exacerbations, disease progression, functional outcomes, and response to therapies (clinical phenotypes) [10]. A unique phenotype, which has similar underlying biologic (physiologic or molecular) mechanisms that define subtypes (referred to as "endotypes") to guide the development of therapy, is sheared between COPD and asthma [11]. In COPD, individual patients with similar degrees of airflow limitation most likely are different in terms of symptoms, exercise capacity, and exacerbation risk. Ever since 2011, Global Initiative for Chronic Obstructive Lung Disease (GOLD) states a multidimensional assessment of patients with COPD that includes two new dimensions: symptoms experienced by the patient and the risk of future exacerbations [1].

Since COPD is heterogeneous, patients with this disease can be stratified according to clinical phenotypes [3, 4, 10]. However, different clinical characteristics are mixed in various proportions in individual patients with COPD. This chapter describes multiple dimensions including clinical, physiologic, imaging, and endotyping dimensions in COPD [9]; moreover, describes effectiveness of corticosteroids with bronchodilators to patients with COPD who have airway eosinophilia and airway hyperresponsiveness as phenotypes in order to search treatable trait for COPD [12].

2. COPD pheotypes

Multiple disease characteristics have been termed COPD phenotypes up until now; and individual patients with COPD can be grouped by phenotypes (phenotypic grouping). These groupings are proposed to determine clusters of patients with common characteristics that relate to clinically meaningful outcomes such as symptoms, exacerbations, response to therapy, and rate of disease progression, or death (stratified medicine) [10, 13]. This more focused definition allows for classifications of patients to distinct prognostic and therapeutic subgroups for both clinical and research purposes as a heterogeneous disease in COPD. The earliest phenotypic classification of COPD was separated into two groups based on physical examination, the "Pink Puffers" and the "Blue Bloaters" [14]. Airflow limitation detected by the routine use of spirometry is insufficient to distinguish COPD from asthma and other airway diseases (chronic bronchitis, pan bronchiolitis, bronchiectasis, etc.). It is especially difficult to distinguish between COPD and asthma. More than 50 years ago, Dutch hypothesis argued that bronchodilator responsiveness was an overlapping feature shared by various forms of obstructive lung diseases, including asthma [15]. In contrast, the British hypothesis argued that bronchodilator responsiveness in patients with COPD was due to concomitant asthma [16]. Hence, multivariable approaches to deal with diseases probably provide relevant information that can characterize different subtypes of COPD. Multiple dimensions for COPD assessment can include clinical, physiologic, imaging, and endotyping dimensions (**Figure 1**) [9]. Data from each dimension support the relevance of specific variables to diagnosis and prognosis for COPD. However, very few and limited combinations of these variables and dimensions have been studied and validated. Therefore, various classification systems for COPD have established taking into phenotypes and endotypes to allow categorization of patients in meaningful methods.

2.1 Clinical dimension

2.1.1 Symptoms

Symptoms (dyspnea, cough, sputum production) and signs (wheezing, prologued exhalation) overlap between COPD and other airway diseases, but with a decline in body mass index (BMI), very little overlap between COPD and asthma. The GOLD Report initially stated a classification system based on reduction in FEV_1 [1]. However, FEV_1 is no clearly associated with symptom severity, functional status, and prognosis [17, 18]. Symptom severity has been shown to be better predictor of mortality than FEV_1 alone in patients with COPD [19]. Health questionnaires such as COPD Assessment Test (CAT) scores and St George Respiratory Questionnaire (SGRQ) scores have been used to understand the relationship between symptoms and quality of life [20]. As an approach includes more variables, a multidimensional grading system including body mass index (BMI), obstruction in the airway (FEV_1), dyspnea, and exercise ability (BODE index) has shown to be better than FEV_1 alone in predicting mortality in patients with COPD [21].

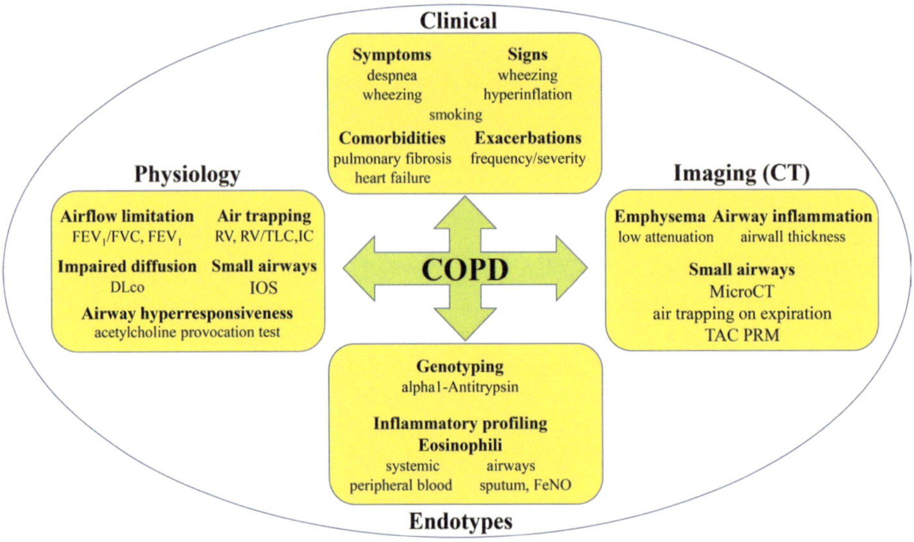

Figure 1.
A Schema of multiple dimensions for assessment of COPD phenotypes. Squares represent dimensions, which is consist of clinical, physiology, imaging CT, and endotypes; and enclose variables with defined or possible relevance to diagnosis, prognosis, or potential therapy in patients with COPD. Illustrated based on ref. [1, 9].

2.1.2 Exacerbations

COPD exacerbations perhaps result in rapid decrease of lung function (FEV_1), deterioration of quality of life, and escalation of healthcare cost [22]. Clinical studies have demonstrated that severe COPD exacerbations are associated with a high mortality [23], and that COPD exacerbations are independent risk factor for morbidity in the disease [24]. Frequent exacerbators are a group of subjects with two or more exacerbations per year [25]. Although recent data suggest that the frequent exacerbator phenotype is quite infrequent in a large cohort study, this phenotype seems to be quite stable over time because the best predictor for exacerbations is history of prior exacerbations [26]. In the recent GOLD Report, the stage of COPD is classified by percentage predicted FEV_1 (Grades I–IV), and separately dyspnea severity and exacerbation history are incorporated into a 2 × 2 grid to form four groups A – D [1]. This assessment approach will guide more precise treatment for individualized patient with COPD. However, this classification is insufficient to seize accurately the heterogeneity of COPD.

During a COPD exacerbation, bacteria, viruses, or both are detected from lower airway secretions in two-thirds of patients, and bacterial/viral coinfection is present in one-fourth [27]. *Hemophilus influenzae, Streptococcus pneumoniae,* and *Moraxella catarrhalis* are isolated as the most common bacterial pathogens during COPD exacerbations. Acquisition of a new bacterial strain precedes exacerbations [28]. Rhino virus is most frequently associated with exacerbations [29], whereas coronavirus, parainfluenza, adenovirus, and influenza virus are less prevalent.

2.1.3 Smoking

Cigarette smokers have a higher prevalence of respiratory symptoms, and impaired lung function, a greater annual rate of decline in FEV_1, and a greater rate of COPD mortality than non-smokers [1]. As shown in the SPIROMICS cohort, respiratory symptoms are present in half of cigarette smokers with preserved lung function. When compared with asymptomatic cigarette smokers, these symptomatic smokers have greater limitation of physical activity, lung function abnormalities (although still within the limits considered as normal), and evidence of airway wall thickening on CT imaging of the chest [30]. Importantly, cigarette smokers with preserved lung function and respiratory symptoms have higher rates of exacerbations than asymptomatic cigarette smokers.

2.1.4 Comorbidity

Patients with COPD have a high prevalence not only of other pulmonary disease (lung cancer, pulmonary hypertension, pulmonary fibrosis, etc.) but also extrapulmonary diseases (cardiovascular diseases, diabetes mellitus, hyperlipidemia, etc.) [31]. This is very important because approximately two-thirds of patients with COPD die from these other diseases, and comorbidities have a significant effect on prognosis or mortality [32, 33]. Recent investigations using network analysis of comorbidities in patients with COPD demonstrate that the presence of hubs of comorbid conditions is highly associated with this disease beyond lung cancer and cardiovascular disease (COPD comorbidity network). Prognosis of patients with COPD is most likely affected by larger number of multiple interlinked morbidities, and their clustering pattern suggests common pathobiological pathways [34].

Combined pulmonary fibrosis and emphysema (CPFE), which is defined by CT imaging of the chest, is closely associated to a history of cigarette smoking. CPFE is characterized by exertional dyspnea, emphysema in the upper lobe, and fibrosis in the lower lobe of the lungs. Patients with CPFE have preserved lung volume (total lung capacity, forced vital capacity) and severely diminished carbon monoxide diffusion capacity of the lung (DLco), moreover, have high prevalence of pulmonary hypertension, and poor prognosis [35]. Survival rate in CPFE is worse than that expected for emphysema without fibrosis; in contrast, survival rate in CPFE is better than that in usual interstitial pneumonia diagnosed by pathological findings. It is still unknown whether the therapy for COPD or pulmonary fibrosis/usual interstitial pneumonia is effective for CPFE. Corticosteroids do not have significant benefit to patients with CPFE.

2.2 Physiological dimension

2.2.1 Airflow limitation

Diagnosis of COPD is based on the physiologic criteria of fixed obstruction in forced expiratory flow (0.7 as cutoff point for FEV_1/FVC ratio); however, the use of a fixed cut point like this probably misclassifies some older patients as developing COPD (more frequent diagnosis of COPD in elderly subjects), compared with the use of a cutoff point derived from the lower limit normal (LLN) for FEV_1/FVC ratio. On the other hand, the use of this fixed cutoff point for FEV_1/FVC ratio results in less frequent diagnosis of COPD in younger adults, compared with that of the LLN. Since the LLN for FEV_1/FVC ratio decreases with age, the accuracy of these diagnostic criteria also should be changed with age [36]. The use of the LLN affects the establishment of early diagnosis for COPD in younger adults. Criterion used in the LLN would be a more desirable parameter that increases the accuracy of diagnosis in this disease. However, those values are dependent on the reference population and are unlikely to accurately reflect the normality of many different ethnic groups. Moreover, there are no longitudinal studies available validating the use of the LLN.

FEV_1 also normally decreases with age, and FEV_1 (% of the predicted value) is used as an indicator for staging of COPD. However, FEV_1 is not always associated with shortness of breath, exercise tolerance, and quality of life [17, 18]. The rate of decrease is probably an important indicator of disease progression in patients with COPD. However, the rate of lung function decrease (a decline of FEV_1) is not also considered for diagnosis or stage classification of this disease. In these approaches using spirometry (the physiologic criteria), first-line medications have been applied consistently in the condition that COPD is once diagnosed without much consideration of possible distinct phenotypes of COPD.

2.2.2 Impaired diffusion

Diffusing capacity derived from DL_{CO} can estimate the potential of gas exchange of the lung [37]. DLco is frequently reduced in patients with established COPD. There is also a subset of cigarette smokers with normal spirometry (FEV_1/FVC ratio > 0.7), who have a low value of DL_{CO}. Decreased DL_{CO} in smokers is pathologically correlated to the destruction of the pulmonary capillary bed, and a low value of DL_{CO} in the context of a normal total lung capacity (TLC) probably indicates alveolar destruction, i.e., emphysema [37, 38] and possibly small airway disease, both of which are components of COPD [39, 40]. Clinical trials have reported a significant correlation between reduced DL_{CO} and emphysema on CT imaging of the chest [41, 42]. Decreased DL_{CO} has also been correlated with dynamic hyperinflation caused by the presence of severe expiratory airflow limitation derived from emphysema and small airway diseases, independent of decreases in FEV_1/FVC or FEV_1 [43]. Moreover, smokers with normal post-bronchodilator FEV_1 but low DL_{CO} have a higher risk of developing COPD with airflow limitation, compared with those with normal post-bronchodilator FEV_1 and normal DL_{CO} [44]. Hence, DL_{CO} measurement is useful for early diagnosis of COPD who are cigarette smokers without airflow limitation. However, this examination is not part of the GOLD criteria and is currently not used as a routine screening tool [45, 46].

2.2.3 Airway trapping

Gas trapping develops in patients with COPD from the early stages of this disease. Gas trapping results in a rise in residual volume (RV), and static hyperinflation, which is an increase in TLC, as airflow limitation worsens. Lung volume such as RV and TLC is impossible to measure by spirometry in the routine use, and these alterations are estimated by body plethysmography and helium dilution lung volume measurement. RV and TLC are probably helpful to characterize the severity of COPD; however, these are not generally used for management of this disease.

Patients with COPD show widely variable exercise capacities. It is recently considered that FEV_1 was a poor predictor of exercise capacity, and that dynamic hyperinflation, which is a concomitant with decreases in inspiratory capacity (IC) and inspiratory reserve volume (IRV), is more closely related to exercise tolerance than FEV_1 [47]. Dynamic hyperinflation is defined as the variable and temporary increase in end expiratory lung volume (EELV) above its baseline value, which occurs when ventilatory demand is acutely increased during exercise [48, 49]. This phenomenon results from gas trapping in the airways. This is usually measured by IC, which accurately reflects changes in EELV provided that TLC remains unaltered. During exercise, in normal subjects, the tidal volume (VT) is markedly increased at the expense of both the IRV and the expiratory reserve volume. In contrast, since airflow is limited and RV is increased in patients with COPD, VT is only a little increased at the expense of their reduced IRV. Therefore, a reduction in IC causes impaired exercise tolerance in patients with this disease. IC can be measured using spirometry, but IC is currently not used as a clinical predictor of exercise capacity.

2.2.4 Small airway obstruction (less than 2 mm diameter)

The current approach to diagnosis and staging of COPD is based on post-bronchodilator FEV_1/FVC ratio, and FEV_1 (% of predicted value) in spirometry, even though this disease is considered generally to begin in the small airways [50]. This area is classically recognized to be the “quiet zone” or “silent zone” because it cannot be easily assessed by means of spirometry alone [51]. The forced oscillation technique, such as impulse oscillation system (IOS) or MostGraph, was been developed to compute the respiratory system impedance that reflects the mechanical properties (resistance and reactance) of the respiratory system [52]. Higher oscillation frequencies (approximately 20 Hz) reflect large airways, and lower oscillation frequencies (<10 Hz) reflect the entire respiratory system, including the small airways. Abnormalities with low oscillation frequencies can be related to disorders in the small airways. However, the forced oscillation technique has not yet been established as clinical test to estimate the small airway function.

Although little is currently known about the clinical relevance of the small airway dysfunction, abnormalities in this area are probably correlated with magnitude of inhaled toxin exposure, severity of respiratory symptoms, response to therapy, presence of systemic inflammation. When the presence of respiratory symptoms in patients is unexplained by using routine clinical evaluation because chest CT and spirometry findings are within the normal range, these results may indicate that small airway disorders develop despite normal airflow on spirometry [53].

2.2.5 Airway hyperresponsiveness

It is classically considered that sensitivity to muscarinic activation is a hallmark of asthma, referred to as airway hyperresponsiveness (AHR). However, recent reports have demonstrated that AHR also develops in as set of COPD [12, 54–56]. Awareness of this paradigm shift is gradually increasing. To evaluate AHR, acetylcholine inhalation challenge is carried out according to the standard method of the Japanese Society of Allergy (Acetylcholine provocation test) [57], which is a modified method reported by Hargreaves and coworkers [58]. The provocation test is ended at a concentration of acetylcholine where FEV_1 is reduced by more than 20% from its baseline value. Threshold values are expressed as a minimal concentration of acetylcholine that reduces FEV_1 by more than 20%. AHR is generally defined as threshold values of less than 8 mg/ml of acetylcholine [56, 59]. Acetylcholine provocation test is most reliable for diagnosis of asthma because this clinical examination has great sensitivity and specificity to diagnosis of asthma [60]. Clinical reports have indicated that AHR is complicated by ~60% or ~ 94% of patients with COPD [61, 62]. Since airway narrowing occurs in COPD because of airflow limitation, exclusion criteria should be established to maintain the accuracy of this provocation test for COPD. Recently, acetylcholine provocation test was carried out for subjects who have FEV1 $\geq$ 70%

predicted values not only to avoid false positives but also to secure safety in this examination [63]. Moreover, the patients with COPD were enrolled in the study and do not have past history of asthma and no clinical features of asthma. As a result, AHR developed in approximate 50% of the patient with COPD excluded asthma [12].

2.3 Imaging dimension

2.3.1 Emphysema

COPD, which is diagnosed in routine use of spirometry, contains both with and without emphysema. Emphysema, which can be easily detected by chest CT, occurs in a significant proportion of cigarette smokers that might not fit the COPD spirometric criteria [64]. Emphysema can be divided into with and without airflow limitation (FEV_1/FVC ratio < 0.7); COPD also can be divided into with and without emphysema. Multiple different phenotypes of emphysema have been described, i.e., centrilobular, panlobular, and paraseptal phenotypes. Some differences are shown among these phenotypes. The centrilobular phenotype is associated with greater smoking history, whereas the panlobular phenotype is associated with reduced body mass index, independent of FEV_1 [65]. Paraseptal emphysema is associated with fewer symptoms and less physiologic impairment. In the analysis of different emphysema patterns based on the Fleischer Society grading system, Kaplan–Meier survival curves demonstrate that patients with absent and trace emphysema have the best survival; those with moderate centrilobular emphysema have intermediate survival; and those with confluent or advanced destructive emphysema have poor survival [66]. However, little is known what determines the distribution of the emphysema. Phenotyping based on the anatomic distribution may result in important therapeutic implications that lung volume reduction surgery may be beneficial to patients with upper-lobe emphysema and low exercise capacity [67].

2.3.2 Small airway

The narrowing and loss of terminal bronchioles occur before the development of emphysema. Assessment of small airway disease is probably useful to identify COPD at an early stage [64, 68]. However, small airways are less than 2 mm in diameter [69]. Because this size falls below the resolution limit of chest CT for direct evaluation, small airways are not imaged directly using routine CT scan. For this reason, novel methods using CT have been devised to evaluate small airways diseases. Micro-CT studies, which are 3D imaging techniques utilizing X-rays to see inside an object, have demonstrated that both total bronchiolar area and the number of small conducting airways are reduced in the early stage [68]. Measures of air trapping on expiratory CT have been used to estimate functional small airway disease, including the ratio of expiratory to inspiratory mean lung density [70, 71], the expiratory to inspiratory relative volume change of voxels with attenuation between 2860 and 2950 HU, and the percentage of voxels below 2856 HU in expiration. However, these imaging techniques have their advantages and limitations. CT total airway count (TAC), which is measured as well as airway inner diameter and wall area using anatomically equivalent airways, reflects the airway-related disease changes in the "quiet" zone (small airways) [72]. A significant decrease in TAC may be observed in early stage of COPD; and that can predict a rapid decline of lung function [72]. The parametric response mapping (PRM), a technique pairing inspiratory and expiratory CT, has been developed to assess small airway diseases. That images to define emphysema (PRM^{emph}) and functional small airways disease (PRM^{fSAD}), a measure of nonemphysematous air trapping [64, 73–76]. These techniques will allow for more accurate diagnosis of individual patients complementing standard clinical examinations to estimate COPD phenotypes. Analysis methods for CT imaging in COPD are making progress to establish novel phenotypes for development of precision medicine according to the results derived from the COPDgene study [75, 76].

Small airways disease occurs in the early stage of COPD and becomes more widespread over time as this disease progresses to more severe. Airway remodeling is observed in this peripheral area in patients with COPD, and pathological findings of that are characterized by goblet cell hyperplasia, mucous gland enlargement, peribronchiolar wall infiltration with inflammatory cells, and bronchiolar smooth muscle hypertrophy [77, 78]. The therapeutic relevance of this phenotype can include use of therapies that allow the small airways to be targeted pharmacologically [79]. However, it is not so easy to estimate accurately diagnosis and treatment outcome in the small airway disease of COPD.

2.4 Endotyping dimension

2.4.1 α_1-Antitrypsin deficiency

It is well known that α_1-antitrypsin is a proteinase inhibitor that protects lung tissue from damage by neutrophil elastase. An imbalance between proteinases and antiproteinases causes destruction of elastin fibers, which affects the elastic recoil of the lung and brings about parenchymal destruction (emphysema). This imbalance between proteinases and antiproteinases seems to be less evident in patients with other forms of emphysema. This condition of α_1-Antitrypsin deficiency is observed less than 5% of patients with COPD and presents in younger subjects compared with the rest of the COPD population [80]. Mutation of the α_1-antitrypsin gene results in a much higher risk of COPD in cigarette smokers and workers exposed to environmental particules. Homozygous α_1-antitrypsin deficiency occurs in 1–4.5% of patients with COPD; in contrast, the heterozygous form occurs in 17.8% of patients with COPD [81]. Previous clinical trial may provide the therapeutic relevance that intravenous augmentation with pooled human α_1-antitrypsin may be beneficial to subjects with severe α_1-antitrypsin deficiency [82].

2.4.2 Inflammatory profiling

It is classically considered that asthma is characterized by eosinophil inflammation in the large airways with Th2 phenotype, om the other hand, that COPD is characterized by initial macrophage, neutrophil, and CD8 lymphocyte inflammation in the small airways [83]. However, it is recently proven that eosinophil and non-TH2 related inflammation is involved not only in the large airways but also the small airways in patients with asthma; on the other hand, eosinophil inflammation is involved in the large airways in patients with COPD. Blood eosinophil counts are increased in COPD patients compared with healthy controls, even when atopic patients are removed from the analysis [84]. This paradigm shift in the approach to this disease is generally recognized. Hence, airway inflammatory profiling is not so useful for differential diagnosis between COPD and asthma since eosinophil inflammation overlaps with these two diseases. The eosinophil count in the peripheral blood may be beneficial as a predictor of the frequency of exacerbations and response to corticosteroid in the management of COPD [85–88]. The increased blood eosinophil numbers may be a reason for increased lung eosinophil numbers observed in a subgroup of COPD patients [89, 90]. According to these reports, it has been assumed all along that blood eosinophilia is a faithful representation of tissue eosinophilia. However, this assumption has not been proven conclusively [91]. The eosinophil count in the peripheral blood does not always correspond to the eosinophil count in the lung tissue. Furthermore, high numbers of blood eosinophils are not associated with frequency of exacerbations [92]. It remains to be solved whether useful blood eosinophil counts are useful as a predictor of the management of COPD. COPD with airway eosinophilia in the tissue probably is a subgroup (phenotype) of this disease, since this phenotype has unique pulmonary and systemic manifestations and a differential response to drugs [87, 88, 93]. This phenotype of COPD probably has a good response to corticosteroids [89]; and sputum examination is probably most reliable as a clinical test to detect eosinophil inflammation in the airways, blood test is not. Blood eosinophilic phenotype was associated with PH. Eosinophilic COPD was associated with higher mPAP and PVR and increased likelihood of PH. More studies are needed to further explore this finding [94].

3. Treatable traits and precision medicine of airway diseases

3.1 Overlap of symptoms and airflow limitation between COPD and asthma

COPD and asthma are the two most prevalent human airway diseases. Although COPD and asthma are pathologically entirely different diseases, it is not so easy to clearly distinguish between these two diseases. In patients with COPD, the initial pathological alterations occur in bronchioles less than 2 mm in diameter ("silent zone" in spirometry). Disorders in the bronchioles are followed by parenchymal remodeling [68], which is different from asthma. On the other hand, disorders in bronchioles probably cause wheezing, which is characteristic to asthma. Clinical manifestations and airflow limitation overlap with COPD and asthma; moreover, eosinophilia and hyperresponsiveness in the airways, which are classically considered to be characteristic of asthma, also overlap with these two diseases. In patients with asthma who have a history of smoking, a differential diagnosis between asthma and COPD can be difficult just in the routine use of spirometry. In these cases that fit the pyrometric criteria for COPD, it may be hard to distinguish clearly between asthma and COPD because of the LLN for FEV_1/FVC ratio and the low incidence (approximately 15%) of COPD in smokers. In patients with COPD who have eosinophilia and hyperresponsiveness in the airways, it is also can be difficult to accurately distinguish between COPD and COPD with asthma even though they have symptoms with variability (cough, dyspnea, wheezing), which are clinical features of asthma, but overlap between COPD and asthma.

3.2 Asthma-COPD overlap

The term asthma-COPD overlap (ACO), which is a phenotype of COPD, is used to identify patients with airway diseases that combine clinical features of both asthma and COPD [8, 95]. However, diagnosis of ACO may be unclear because COPD and asthma may be unclear because these two diseases are heterogeneous. It is also unclear to accurately distinguish between ACO and COPD with eosinophilia in peripheral blood. There is still disagreement with ACO; and the concept of ACO remains quite controversial [11, 96]. ACO is diagnosed for a patient who has characteristic of COPD, namely persistent airflow limitation as well as features of asthma [8]. Features of asthma develop in between approximately 15% of patients with COPD as well [8, 97]. ACO is not a single uniform entity but consists of multiple sub-phenotypes, such as asthma with irreversible airway obstruction due to structural changes, or smoke or predominantly neutrophilic inflammation, and COPD with eosinophilic inflammation [97]. It is generally considered that patients with ACO appear to have more symptoms, more frequent exacerbations, increased risk of hospitalization, and a worse quality of life [98]; on the other hand, patients with ACO appear to have a lower mortality [95]. The identification of ACO is important because corticosteroids are beneficial to patients with ACO, regardless of FEV_1 or exacerbation frequency [99]. The responsiveness to corticosteroids is due to feature of asthma in ACO.

3.3 Airway eosinophilia and airway hyperresponsiveness as phenotypes of COPD

Since airway eosinophilia and AHR overlap between COPD and asthma, the differential diagnosis between COPD, asthma, and ACO can be unclear in cases with eosinophilia and AHR in the airways. It also still unclear to distinguish accurately between eosinophilic COPD and COPD with asthma [100]. A previous report that examined airway eosinophilic inflammation using sputum induction and examined AHR using methacholine provocation test in 21 cases of COPD has indicated that 41.4% had AHR, 31.0% had increased sputum eosinophils, and that cases with AHR had higher sputum eosinophils than cases without AHR and those with sputum eosinophils more than 3% had more exacerbations in the previous year [55]. In another study, 203 patients with COPD who have no symptoms and past history related to asthma were enrolled to examine role of eosinophilic inflammation and AHR in the airways as phenotypes of COPD [12]. These subjects were diagnosed as COPD based on lung function test and smoking history. Eosinophils in the sputum were observed in 65 (50.4%) of 129 subjects using qualitative analysis; in contrast, lower grade (more than 0%, less than 3%) and higher grade (3% or more) were observed in 15 (20.3%) and 25 (33.8%) of 74 subjects using quantitative analysis [12]. Exacerbations occurred much more frequently in lower-grade airway eosinophilia without inhaled corticosteroid than in higher-grade airway eosinophilia with inhaled corticosteroid [12]. Regulation of airway eosinophilia is associated with a reduction in exacerbations of COPD (**Figure 2**) [101]. AHR developed in 46.9% of these subjects with sputum eosinophils; but grade of airway eosinophilia was not associated with development of AHR. AHR also significantly increased frequency of exacerbations in COPD with both lower and higher grade in airway eosinophilia [12]. This clinical report demonstrates that airway eosinophilia and AHR cause in COPD, independent of asthma, and that these phenotypes of COPD are closely related to symptom stability (exacerbations). Moreover, AHR is associated with mortality in COPD [102–104]. These essential results derived from these clinical studies are summarized in **Figures 2**, **3** and **Table 1**.

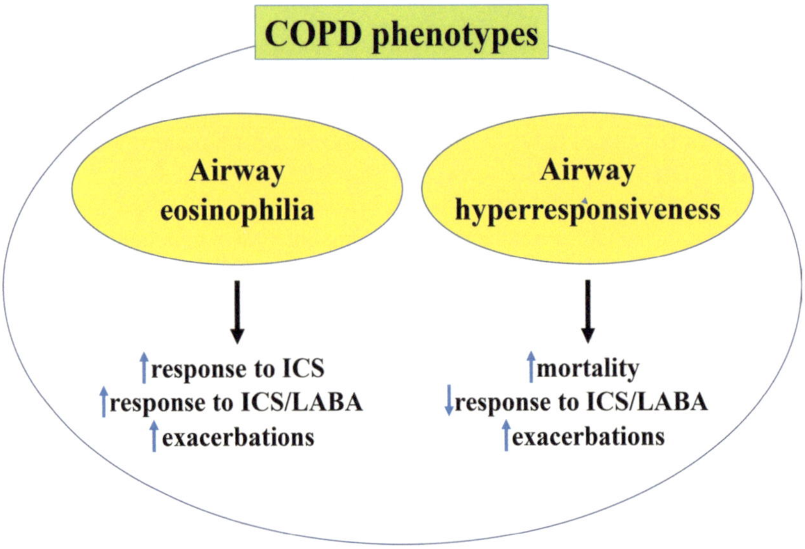

Figure 2.
Clinical characteristics caused by airway eosinophilia and airway hyperresponsiveness as phenotypes of COPD. Illustrated based on ref. [12, 55, 89, 101–109].

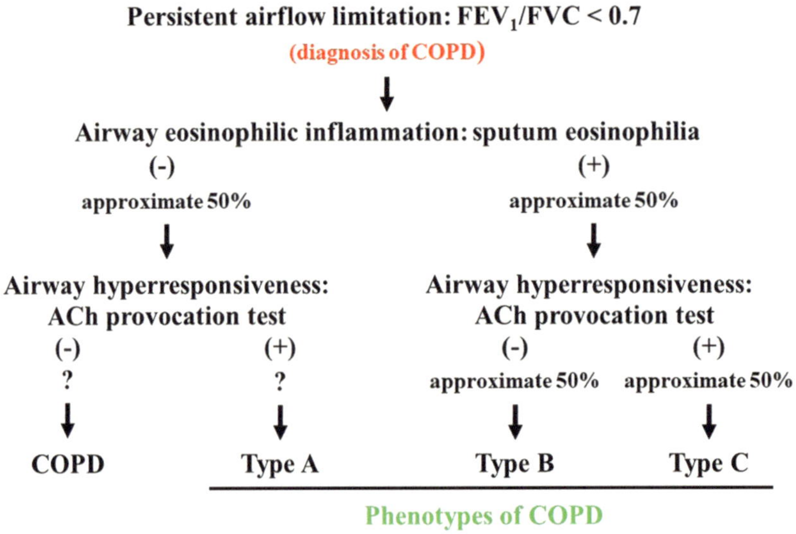

Figure 3.
Phenotypes of COPD classified into airway eosinophilia and airway hyperresponsiveness. Illustrated based on ref. [12, 55].

3.4 Phenotypes and response to corticosteroids with bronchodilators

COPD with peripheral blood eosinophilia may have a particularly favorable response to inhaled corticosteroid (ICS)/long-acting β_2-adrenergic agonist (LABA) therapy, perhaps because of the inflammation profiling that responds well to corticosteroids. However, prospective studies are required to evaluate the role of blood

	Phenotypes of COPD		
Treatable traits	**Type A**	**Type B**	**Type C**
$FEV_1/FVC < 0.7$	+	+	+
Sputum eosinophils	−	+	+
ACh provocation PC_{20} < 5000 μg/mL	+	−	+
Stability and therapy	**Type A**	**Type B**	**Type C**
Frequency of exacerbations	+	++	+++
Response to ICS with LABA	unknown	more potent	less potent

Table 1.
Effects of airway eosinophilia and airway hyperresponsiveness as treatable traits on the management of COPD. Illustrated based on refs. [12, 55].

eosinophils as a biomarker of inhaled therapy response in COPD [110]. Eosinophil counts in the peripheral blood are not always associated with those in the airways. For this reason, patients with COPD who have sputum eosinophilia were enrolled to examine involvement of eosinophilic inflammation in response to corticosteroids and LABA [12, 55, 105, 106]. Inhaled indacaterol (a LABA) caused a greater increase in FEV_1 [107] and IC [108] in these patients than those shown in other previous reports. Addition of inhaled ciclesonide (a corticosteroid) to indacaterol caused much higher increases in FEV_1 and IC, and values of CAT score and frequency of on demand use of procaterol (a short-acting β_2-adrenergic agonist) were markedly reduced (**Table 1**) [12]. These results indicate that not only ICS but also LABA is effective in improving lung function, symptoms, and quality of life in COPD with airway eosinophilia [109]. Since airway inflammation induced by neutrophils and oxidative stress may be the main pathogenesis of COPD, ICS is generally considered to be not so beneficial to this disease. However, ICS/LABA is beneficial to airway eosinophilic inflammation in COPD, similar to that in asthma. Indacaterol, a strong partial β_2-adrenergic agonist, is probably effective for COPD because of higher values of its intrinsic efficacy close to a full agonist [111–115]. In these patients with COPD who have sputum eosinophilia, there was no deference in response to indacaterol for FEV_1 and IC between these subjects with and without AHR; in contrast, addition to ciclesonide caused greater increases in FEV_1 and IC in these subjects without AHR than in these subjects with AHR [12]. However, mechanisms underlining this reduced responsiveness to corticosteroids in COPD with AHR have not been investigated in detail. Therefore, airway eosinophilia and AHR affect symptom suitability (exacerbations) and responsiveness to corticosteroids and β_2-adrenergic agonists in COPD (**Table 1**, **Figure 2**).

4. Conclusions

Although it is generally considered that COPD has heterogeneity, COPD is currently diagnosed based on physiologic criteria using spirometry. Hence, individual patients with COPD should be classified by distinct phenotypes (stratified medicine). Research for characterization of different subtypes COPD has been conducted on according to multivariable approaches to address disease using multiple dimensions including clinical, physiologic, imaging, and endotyping [1, 9] (**Figure 1**). However, possible distinct phenotypes have been not yet established up to today. Recently,

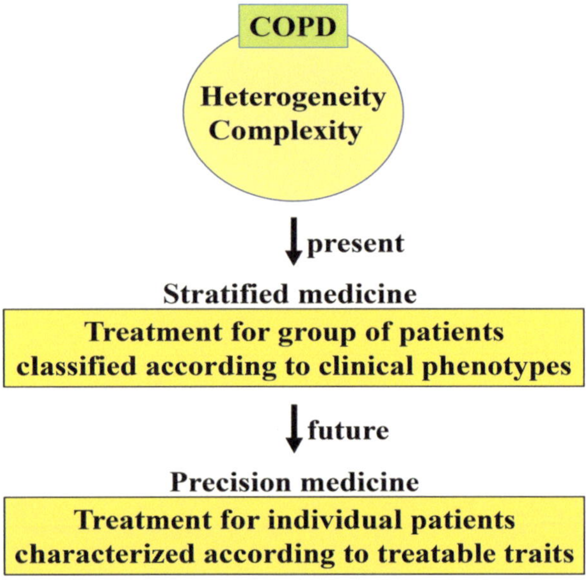

Figure 4.
A direction to aim for the management of COPD. Precision medicine of personalized medicine is suitable for a heterogeneous disease. Illustrated based on refs. [1, 3, 5].

precision medicine due to treatable trait has been proposed as aimed treatment for COPD in near future [3–5] (**Figure 4**). It is defined as treatments targeted to the needs of individual patients based on genetic, biomarker, phenotypic, or psychosocial characteristics that distinguish a given patient from other patients with similar clinical presentations (personalized medicine) [116–119].

Conflict of interest

Hiroaki Kume: none.
Ryuki Yamada: none.
Yuki Sato: none.

Author details

Hiroaki Kume*, Ryuki Yamada and Yuki Sato
Department of Infectious Diseases and Respiratory Medicine, Fukushima Medical University Aizu Medical Center, Fukushima, Japan

*Address all correspondence to: h-kume@fmu.ac.jp

References

[1] Global Initiative for Chronic Obstructive Lung Disease. Global strategy for prevention, diagnosis and management of COPD. 2022. Available online: https://goldcopd.org/

[2] Spurzem JR, Rennard SI. Pathogenesis of COPD. Seminars in Respiratory and Critical Care Medicine. 2005;**26**(2):142-153. DOI: 10.1055/s-2005-869535

[3] Agusti A. The path to personalised medicine in COPD. Thorax. 2014;**69**(9):857-864. DOI: 10.1136/thoraxjnl-2014-205507

[4] Agusti A, Bel E, Thomas M, et al. Treatable traits: Toward precision medicine of chronic airway diseases. The European Respiratory Journal. 2016;**47**(2):410-419. DOI: 10.1183/13993003.01359-2015

[5] Agustí A, Bafadhel M, Beasley R, et al. Precision medicine in airway diseases: Moving to clinical practice. The European Respiratory Journal. 2017;**50**(4):1701655. DOI: 10.1183/13993003.01655-2017

[6] Hogg JC. Pathophysiology of airflow limitation in chronic obstructive pulmonary disease. Lancet. 2004;**364**(9435):701

[7] Standards for diagnosis and care of patients with chronic obstructive lung disease. American Journal of Respiratory and Critical Care Medicine. 1995;**152**:S77-S121

[8] Gibson PG, McDonald VM. Asthma-COPD overlap 2015: Now we are six. Thorax. 2015;**70**(7):683-691. DOI: 10.1136/thoraxjnl-2014-206740

[9] Segal LN, Martinez FJ. Chronic obstructive pulmonary disease subpopulations and phenotyping. The Journal of Allergy and Clinical Immunology. 2018;**141**:961-1971. DOI: 10.1016/j.jaci.2018.02.035

[10] Han MK, Agusti A, Calverley PM, et al. Chronic obstructive pulmonary disease phenotypes: The future of COPD. American Journal of Respiratory and Critical Care Medicine. 2010;**182**:598-604. DOI: 10.1164/rccm.200912-1843CC

[11] Woodruff PG, van den Berge M, Boucher RC, et al. American Thoracic Society/National Heart, Lung, and Blood Institute asthma-chronic obstructive pulmonary disease overlap workshop report. American Journal of Respiratory and Critical Care Medicine. 2017;**196**:375-381. DOI: 10.1164/rccm.201705-0973WS

[12] Kume H, Hojo M, Hashimoto N. Eosinophil inflammation and hyperresponsiveness in the airways as phenotypes of COPD, and usefulness of inhaled Glucocorticosteroids. Frontiers in Pharmacology. 2019;**10**:765. DOI: 10.3389/fphar.2019.00765

[13] Agustí A. Phenotypes and disease characterization in chronic obstructive pulmonary disease. Toward the extinction of phenotypes? Annals of the American Thoracic Society. 2013;**10**(Suppl):S125-S130. DOI: 10.1513/AnnalsATS.201303-055AW

[14] Dornhorst AC. Respiratory insufficiency. Lancet. 1955;**268**:1185-1187

[15] Barnes PJ. Against the Dutch hypothesis: Asthma and chronic obstructive pulmonary disease are distinct diseases. American Journal of Respiratory and Critical Care Medicine. 2006;**174**:240-243

[16] Kraft M. Asthma and chronic obstructive pulmonary disease exhibit common origins in any country! American Journal of Respiratory and Critical Care Medicine. 2006;**174**:238-240

[17] Wolkove N, Dajczman E, Colacone A, et al. The relationship between pulmonary function and dyspnea in obstructive lung disease. Chest. 1989;**96**:1247-1251. DOI: 10.1378/chest.96.6.1247

[18] Jones P, Miravitlles M, van der Molen T, et al. Beyond FEV_1 in COPD: A review of patient-reported outcomes and their measurement. International Journal of Chronic Obstructive Pulmonary Disease. 2012;**7**:697-709. DOI: 10.2147/COPD.S32675

[19] Nishimura K, Izumi T, Tsukino M, et al. Dyspnea is a better predictor of 5-year survival than airway obstruction in patients with COPD. Chest. 2002;**121**:1434-1440. DOI: 10.1378/chest.121.5.1434

[20] Jones PW, Quirk FH, Baveystock CM, et al. A self-complete measure of health status for chronic airflow limitation. The St. George's Respiratory Questionnaire. The American Review of Respiratory Disease. 1992;**145**:1321-1337. DOI: 10.1164/ajrccm/145.6.1321

[21] Celli BR, Cote CG, Lareau SC, et al. Predictors of survival in COPD: More than just the FEV1. Respiratory Medicine. 2008;**102**(Suppl 1):S27-S35. DOI: 10.1016/S0954-6111(08)70005-2

[22] Anzueto A. Impact of exacerbations on COPD. European Respiratory Review. 2010;**19**:113-118. DOI: 10.1183/09059180.00002610

[23] Soler-Cataluña JJ, Martínez-García MA, Román Sánchez P, et al. Severe acute exacerbations and mortality in patients with chronic obstructive pulmonary disease. Thorax. 2005;**60**:925-931. DOI: 10.1136/thx.2005.040527

[24] Schmidt SA, Johansen MB, Olsen M, et al. The impact of exacerbation frequency on mortality following acute exacerbations of COPD: A registry-based cohort study. BMJ Open. 2014;**4**:e006720. DOI: 10.1136/bmjopen-2014-006720

[25] Hurst JR, Vestbo J, Anzueto A, et al. Susceptibility to exacerbation in chronic obstructive pulmonary disease. The New England Journal of Medicine. 2010;**363**:1128-1138. DOI: 10.1056/NEJMoa0909883

[26] Han MK, Quibrera PM, Carretta EE, et al. Frequency of exacerbations in patients with chronic obstructive pulmonary disease: An analysis of the SPIROMICS cohort. The Lancet Respiratory Medicine. 2017;**5**:619-626. DOI: 10.1016/S2213-2600(17)30207-2

[27] Monsó E, Ruiz J, Rosell A, Manterola J, et al. Bacterial infection in chronic obstructive pulmonary disease. A study of stable and exacerbated outpatients using the protected specimen brush. American Journal of Respiratory and Critical Care Medicine. 1995;**152**:1316-1320. DOI: 10.1164/ajrccm.152.4.7551388

[28] Sethi S, Sethi R, Eschberger K, et al. Airway bacterial concentrations and exacerbations of chronic obstructive pulmonary disease. American Journal of Respiratory and Critical Care Medicine. 2007;**176**:356-361. DOI: 10.1164/rccm.200703-417OC

[29] Seemungal T, Harper-Owen R, Bhowmik A, et al. Respiratory viruses, symptoms, and inflammatory markers in acute exacerbations and stable chronic obstructive pulmonary disease. American Journal of Respiratory and Critical

Care Medicine. 2001;**164**:1618-1623. DOI: 10.1164/ajrccm.164.9.2105011

[30] Woodruff PG, Barr RG, Bleecker E, et al. Clinical significance of symptoms in smokers with preserved pulmonary function. The New England Journal of Medicine. 2016;**374**:1811-1821. DOI: 10.1056/NEJMoa1505971

[31] Schnell K, Weiss CO, Lee T, et al. The prevalence of clinically-relevant comorbid conditions in patients with physician-diagnosed COPD: A cross-sectional study using data from NHANES 1999-2008. BMC Pulmonary Medicine. 2012;**12**:26. DOI: 10.1186/1471-2466-12-26

[32] Crisafulli E, Costi S, Luppi F, et al. Role of comorbidities in a cohort of patients with COPD undergoing pulmonary rehabilitation. Thorax. 2008;**63**:487-492. DOI: 10.1136/thx.2007.086371

[33] Divo MJ, Cote C, de Torres JP, et al. Comorbidities and risk of mortality in patients with chronic obstructive pulmonary disease. American Journal of Respiratory and Critical Care Medicine. 2012;**186**:155-161. DOI: 10.1164/rccm.201201-0034OC

[34] Divo MJ, Casanova C, Marin JM, et al. COPD comorbidities network. The European Respiratory Journal. 2015;**46**:640-650. DOI: 10.1183/09031936.00171614

[35] Cottin V, Nunes H, Brillet PY, et al. Combined pulmonary fibrosis and emphysema: A distinct underrecognised entity. The European Respiratory Journal. 2005;**26**:586-593. DOI: 10.1183/09031936.05.00021005

[36] Cerveri I, Corsico AG, Accordini S, et al. Underestimation of airflow obstruction among young adults using $FEV_1/FVC < 70\%$ as a fixed cut-off: A longitudinal evaluation of clinical and functional outcomes. Thorax. 2008;**63**:1040-1045. DOI: 10.1136/thx.2008.095554

[37] Crapo RO, Jensen RL, Wanger JS. Single-breath carbon monoxide diffusing capacity. Clinics in Chest Medicine. 2001;**22**:637-649. DOI: 10.1016/s0272-5231(05)70057-5

[38] Hogg JC. Pathophysiology of airflow limitation in chronic obstructive pulmonary disease. Lancet. 2004;**364**:709-721. DOI: 10.1016/S0140-6736(04)16900-6

[39] Klein JS, Gamsu G, Webb WR, et al. High-resolution CT diagnosis of emphysema in symptomatic patients with normal chest radiographs and isolated low diffusing capacity. Radiology. 1992;**182**:817-821. DOI: 10.1148/radiology.182.3.1535900

[40] Matheson MC, Raven J, Johns DP, et al. Associations between reduced diffusing capacity and airflow obstruction in community-based subjects. Respiratory Medicine. 2007;**101**:1730-1737. DOI: 10.1016/j.rmed.2007.02.020

[41] Gurney JW, Jones KK, Robbins RA, et al. Regional distribution of emphysema: Correlation of high-resolution CT with pulmonary function tests in unselected smokers. Radiology. 1992;**183**:457-463. DOI: 10.1148/radiology.183.2.1561350

[42] Coxson HO, Rogers RM, Whittall KP, et al. A quantification of the lung surface area in emphysema using computed tomography. American Journal of Respiratory and Critical Care Medicine. 1999;**159**:851-856. DOI: 10.1164/ajrccm.159.3.9805067

[43] Gelb AF, Zamel N, Hogg JC, et al. Pseudophysiologic emphysema resulting

from severe small-airways disease. American Journal of Respiratory and Critical Care Medicine. 1998;**158**:815-819. DOI: 10.1164/ajrccm.158.3.9801045

[44] Harvey BG, Strulovici-Barel Y, Kaner RJ, et al. Risk of COPD with obstruction in active smokers with normal spirometry and reduced diffusion capacity. The European Respiratory Journal. 2015;**46**:1589-1597. DOI: 10.1183/13993003.02377-2014

[45] Macintyre N, Crapo RO, Viegi G, et al. Standardisation of the single-breath determination of carbon monoxide uptake in the lung. The European Respiratory Journal. 2005;**26**:720-735. DOI: 10.1183/09031936.05.00034905

[46] Rabe KF, Hurd S, Anzueto A, et al. Global initiative for chronic obstructive lung disease. Global strategy for the diagnosis, management, and prevention of chronic obstructive pulmonary disease: GOLD executive summary. American Journal of Respiratory and Critical Care Medicine. 2007;**176**:532-555

[47] Diaz O, Villafranca C, Ghezzo H, et al. Role of inspiratory capacity on exercise tolerance in COPD patients with and without tidal expiratory flow limitation at rest. The European Respiratory Journal. 2000;**16**:269-275. DOI: 10.1034/j.1399-3003.2000.16b14.x

[48] O'Donnell DE, Laveneziana P. Physiology and consequences of lung hyperinflation in COPD. European Respiratory Review. 2006;**15**:61-67. DOI: 10.1183/09059180.00010002

[49] Guenette JA, Webb KA, O'Donnell DE. Does dynamic hyperinflation contribute to dyspnoea during exercise in patients with COPD? The European Respiratory Journal. 2012;**40**:322-329. DOI: 10.1183/09031936.00157711

[50] Hogg JC, Paré PD, Hackett TL. The contribution of small airway obstruction to the pathogenesis of chronic obstructive pulmonary disease. Physiological Reviews. 2017;**97**:529-552. DOI: 10.1152/physrev.00025.2015

[51] Macklem PT, Mead J. Resistance of central and peripheral airways measured by a retrograde catheter. Journal of Applied Physiology. 1967;**22**:395-401. DOI: 10.1152/jappl.1967.22.3.395

[52] Dubois AB, Brody AW, Lewis DH, et al. Oscillation mechanics of lungs and chest in man. Journal of Applied Physiology. 1956;**8**:587-594. DOI: 10.1152/jappl.1956.8.6.587

[53] Berger KI, Kalish S, Shao Y, er al. Isolated small airway reactivity during bronchoprovocation as a mechanism for respiratory symptoms in WTC dust-exposed community members. American Journal of Industrial Medicine. 2016;**59**:767-776. DOI: 10.1002/ajim.22639

[54] Tashkin DP, Altose MD, Connett JE, et al. Methacholine reactivity predicts changes in lung function over time in smokers with early chronic obstructive pulmonary disease. The Lung Health Study Research Group. American Journal of Respiratory and Critical Care Medicine. 1996;**153**:1802-1811. DOI: 10.1164/ajrccm.153.6.8665038

[55] Zanini A, Cherubino F, Zampogna E, et al. Bronchial hyperresponsiveness, airway inflammation, and reversibility in patients with chronic obstructive pulmonary disease. International Journal of Chronic Obstructive Pulmonary Disease. 2015;**10**:1155-1161. DOI: 10.2147/COPD.S80992

[56] Tkacova R, Dai DLY, Vonk JM, et al. Airway hyperresponsiveness in chronic obstructive pulmonary disease:

A marker of asthma-chronic obstructive pulmonary disease overlap syndrome? The Journal of Allergy and Clinical Immunology. 2016;**138**:1571-1579.e10. DOI: 10.1016/j.jaci.2016.04.022

[57] Makino S, Ikemori R, Fukuda T, et al. Clinical evaluation of standard method of acetylcholine inhalation test in bronchial asthma. Arerugi. 1984;**33**:167-175

[58] Hargreave FE, Ryan G, Thomson NC, et al. Bronchial responsiveness to histamine or methacholine in asthma: Measurement and clinical significance. The Journal of Allergy and Clinical Immunology. 1981;**68**:347-355. DOI: 10.1016/0091-6749(81)90132-9

[59] De Meer G, Heederik D, Postma DS. Bronchial responsiveness to adenosine 5′-monophosphate (AMP) and methacholine differ in their relationship with airway allergy and baseline FEV_1. American Journal of Respiratory and Critical Care Medicine. 2002;**165**:327-331. DOI: 10.1164/ajrccm.165.3.2104066

[60] Sumino K, Sugar EA, Irvin CG, et al. Methacholine challenge test: Diagnostic characteristics in asthmatic patients receiving controller medications. The Journal of Allergy and Clinical Immunology. 2012;**130**:69-75.e6. DOI: 10.1016/j.jaci.2012.02.025

[61] Tashkin DP, Altose MD, Bleecker ER, et al. The lung health study: Airway responsiveness to inhaled methacholine in smokers with mild to moderate airflow limitation. The American Review of Respiratory Disease. 1992;**145**:301-310. DOI: 10.1164/ajrccm/145.2_Pt_1.301

[62] van den Berge M, Vonk JM, Gosman M, et al. Clinical and inflammatory determinants of bronchial hyperresponsiveness in COPD. The European Respiratory Journal. 2012;**40**:1098-1105. DOI: 10.1183/09031936.00169711

[63] Brutsche MH, Downs SH, Schindler C, et al. Bronchial hyperresponsiveness and the development of asthma and COPD in asymptomatic individuals: SAPALDIA cohort study. Thorax. 2006;**61**:671-677. DOI: 10.1136/thx.2005.052241

[64] Labaki WW, Martinez CH, Martinez FJ, et al. The role of chest computed tomography in the evaluation and Management of the Patient with chronic obstructive pulmonary disease. American Journal of Respiratory and Critical Care Medicine. 2017;**196**:1372-1379. DOI: 10.1164/rccm.201703-0451PP

[65] Smith BM, Austin JH, Newell JD Jr, et al. Pulmonary emphysema subtypes on computed tomography. The American Journal of Medicine. 2014;**127**(94):e7-e23. DOI: 10.1016/j.amjmed.2013.09.020

[66] Lynch DA, Moore CM, Wilson C, et al. Genetic epidemiology of COPD (COPDGene) investigators. CT-based visual classification of emphysema: Association with mortality in the COPDGene study. Radiology. 2018;**288**:859-866. DOI: 10.1148/radiol.2018172294

[67] Fishman A, Martinez F, Naunheim K, et al. A randomized trial comparing lung-volume-reduction surgery with medical therapy for severe emphysema. The New England Journal of Medicine. 2003;**348**:2059-2073. DOI: 10.1056/NEJMoa030287

[68] McDonough JE, Yuan R, Suzuki M, et al. Small-airway obstruction and emphysema in chronic obstructive pulmonary disease. The New England Journal of Medicine. 2011;**365**:1567-1575. DOI: 10.1056/NEJMoa1106955

[69] Hogg JC, Macklem PT, Thurlbeck WM. Site and nature of

airway obstruction in chronic obstructive lung disease. The New England Journal of Medicine. 1968;**278**:1355-1360. DOI: 10.1056/NEJM196806202782501

[70] Eda S, Kubo K, Fujimoto K, et al. The relations between expiratory chest CT using helical CT and pulmonary function tests in emphysema. American Journal of Respiratory and Critical Care Medicine. 1997;**155**:1290-1294. DOI: 10.1164/ajrccm.155.4.9105069

[71] O'Donnell RA, Peebles C, Ward JA, et al. Relationship between peripheral airway dysfunction, airway obstruction, and neutrophilic inflammation in COPD. Thorax. 2004;**59**:837-842. DOI: 10.1136/thx.2003.019349

[72] Kirby M, Tanabe N, Tan WC, et al. Total airway count on computed tomography and the risk of chronic obstructive pulmonary disease progression. Findings from a population-based study. American Journal of Respiratory and Critical Care Medicine. 2018;**197**:56-65. DOI: 10.1164/rccm.201704-0692OC

[73] Galbán CJ, Han MK, Boes JL, et al. Computed tomography-based biomarker provides unique signature for diagnosis of COPD phenotypes and disease progression. Nature Medicine. 2012;**18**:1711-1715. DOI: 10.1038/nm.2971

[74] Bhatt SP, Soler X, Wang X, et al. Association between functional small airway disease and FEV1 decline in chronic obstructive pulmonary disease. American Journal of Respiratory and Critical Care Medicine. 2016;**194**:178-184. DOI: 10.1164/rccm.201511-2219OC

[75] Bhatt SP, Washko GR, Hoffman EA, et al. Imaging advances in chronic obstructive pulmonary disease. Insights from the genetic epidemiology of chronic obstructive pulmonary disease (COPDGene) study. American Journal of Respiratory and Critical Care Medicine. 2019;**199**:286-301. DOI: 10.1164/rccm.201807-1351SO

[76] Castaldi PJ, Boueiz A, Yun J, et al. Machine learning characterization of COPD subtypes: Insights from the COPDGene study. Chest. 2020;**157**:1147-1157. DOI: 10.1016/j.chest.2019.11.039

[77] Maestrelli P, Saetta M, Mapp CE, et al. Remodeling in response to infection and injury. Airway inflammation and hypersecretion of mucus in smoking subjects with chronic obstructive pulmonary disease. American Journal of Respiratory and Critical Care Medicine. 2001;**164**:S76-S80. DOI: 10.1164/ajrccm.164.supplement_2.2106067

[78] Hogg JC, Timens W. The pathology of chronic obstructive pulmonary disease. Annual Review of Pathology. 2009;**4**:435-459. DOI: 10.1146/annurev.pathol.4.110807.092145

[79] Singh D, Nicolini G, Bindi E, et al. Extrafine beclomethasone/formoterol compared to fluticasone/salmeterol combination therapy in COPD. BMC Pulmonary Medicine. 2014;**14**:43. DOI: 10.1186/1471-2466-14-43

[80] Turino GM, Seniorrm GBD, Keller S, et al. Serum elastase inhibitor deficiency and alpha 1-antitrypsin deficiency in patients with obstructive emphysema. Science. 1969;**165**:709-711. DOI: 10.1126/science.165.3894.709

[81] American Thoracic Society/European Respiratory Society statement: Standards for the diagnosis and management of individuals with alpha-1 antitrypsin deficiency. American Thoracic Society; European Respiratory Society. American Journal of Respiratory and Critical Care Medicine. 2003;**168**:818-900. DOI: 10.1164/rccm.168.7.818

[82] Chapman KR, Burdon JG, Piitulainen E, et al. Intravenous augmentation treatment and lung density in severe α1 antitrypsin deficiency (RAPID): A randomised, double-blind, placebo-controlled trial. Lancet. 2015;**386**:360-368. DOI: 10.1016/S0140-6736(15)60860-1

[83] Barnes PJ. Immunology of asthma and chronic obstructive pulmonary disease. Nature Reviews. Immunology. 2008;**8**:183-192. DOI: 10.1038/nri2254

[84] Kolsum U, Southworth T, Jackson N, et al. Blood eosinophil counts in COPD patients compared to controls. The European Respiratory Journal. 2019;**54**:1900633. DOI: 10.1183/13993003.00633-2019

[85] Bafadhel M, McKenna S, Terry S, et al. Acute exacerbations of chronic obstructive pulmonary disease: Identification of biologic clusters and their biomarkers. American Journal of Respiratory and Critical Care Medicine. 2011;**184**:662-671. DOI: 10.1164/rccm.201104-0597OC

[86] Bafadhel M, McKenna S, Terry S, Brightling CE, et al. Blood eosinophils to direct corticosteroid treatment of exacerbations of chronic obstructive pulmonary disease: A randomized placebo-controlled trial. American Journal of Respiratory and Critical Care Medicine. 2012;**186**:48-55. DOI: 10.1164/rccm.201108-1553OC

[87] Pascoe S, Locantore N, Dransfield MT, et al. Blood eosinophil counts as markers of response to inhaled corticosteroids in COPD? The Lancet Respiratory Medicine. 2015;**3**:e27. DOI: 10.1016/S2213-2600(15)00259-3

[88] Siddiqui SH, Guasconi A, Vestbo J, et al. Blood eosinophils: A biomarker of response to Extrafine beclomethasone/formoterol in chronic obstructive pulmonary disease. American Journal of Respiratory and Critical Care Medicine. 2015;**192**:523-525. DOI: 10.1164/rccm.201502-0235LE

[89] Brightling CE, McKenna S, Hargadon B, et al. Sputum eosinophilia and the short term response to inhaled mometasone in chronic obstructive pulmonary disease. Thorax. 2005;**60**:193-198. DOI: 10.1136/thx.2004.032516

[90] Kolsum U, Donaldson GC, Singh R, et al. Blood and sputum eosinophils in COPD; relationship with bacterial load. Respiratory Research. 2017;**18**:88. DOI: 10.1186/s12931-017-0570-5

[91] Dodd PJ, Gardiner E, Coghlan R, et al. Burden of childhood tuberculosis in 22 high-burden countries: A mathematical modelling study. The Lancet Global Health. 2014;**2**:e453-e459. DOI: 10.1016/S2214-109X(14)70245-1

[92] Turato G, Semenzato U, Bazzan E, et al. Blood eosinophilia neither reflects tissue eosinophils nor worsens clinical outcomes in chronic obstructive pulmonary disease. American Journal of Respiratory and Critical Care Medicine. 2018;**197**:1216-1219. DOI: 10.1164/rccm.201708-1684LE

[93] Bafadhel M, Peterson S, De Blas MA, et al. Predictors of exacerbation risk and response to budesonide in patients with chronic obstructive pulmonary disease: A post-hoc analysis of three randomised trials. The Lancet Respiratory Medicine. 2018;**6**:117-126. DOI: 10.1016/S2213-2600(18)30006-7

[94] Alzghoul BN, As Sayaideh M, Moreno BF, et al. Pulmonary hypertension in eosinophilic versus noneosinophilic COPD. ERJ Open Research. 2021;(7):00772-02020

[95] Cosio BG, Soriano JB, López-Campos JL, et al. Defining the

asthma-COPD overlap syndrome in a COPD cohort. Chest. 2016;**149**:45-52. DOI: 10.1378/chest.15-1055

[96] Sin DD, Miravitlles M, Mannino DM, et al. What is asthma-COPD overlap syndrome? Towards a consensus definition from a round table discussion. The European Respiratory Journal. 2016;**48**:664-673. DOI: 10.1183/13993003.00436-2016

[97] Barnes PJ. Asthma-COPD overlap. Chest. 2016;**149**:7-8. DOI: 10.1016/j.chest.2015.08.017

[98] Kauppi P, Kupiainen H, Lindqvist A, et al. Overlap syndrome of asthma and COPD predicts low quality of life. The Journal of Asthma. 2011;**48**:279-285. DOI: 10.3109/02770903.2011.555576

[99] Barnes PJ. Therapeutic approaches to asthma-chronic obstructive pulmonary disease overlap syndromes. The Journal of Allergy and Clinical Immunology. 2015;**136**:531-545. DOI: 10.1016/j.jaci.2015.05.052

[100] Kolsum U, Ravi A, Hitchen P, et al. Clinical characteristics of eosinophilic COPD versus COPD patients with a history of asthma. Respiratory Research. 2017;**18**:73. DOI: 10.1186/s12931-017-0559-0

[101] Siva R, Green RH, Brightling CE, et al. Eosinophilic airway inflammation and exacerbations of COPD: A randomised controlled trial. The European Respiratory Journal. 2007;**29**:906-913. DOI: 10.1183/09031936.00146306

[102] Hospers JJ, Postma DS, Rijcken B, Weiss ST, Schouten JP. Histamine airway hyper-responsiveness and mortality from chronic obstructive pulmonary disease: A cohort study. Lancet. 2000;**356**:1313-1317. DOI: 10.1016/S0140-6736(00)02815-4

[103] Scichilone N, Battaglia S, La Sala A, Bellia V. Clinical implications of airway hyperresponsiveness in COPD. International Journal of Chronic Obstructive Pulmonary Disease. 2006;**1**:49-60. DOI: 10.2147/copd.2006.1.1.49

[104] Teferra AA, Vonk JM, Boezen HM. Longitudinal changes in airway hyperresponsiveness and COPD mortality. The European Respiratory Journal. 2020;**55**:1901378. DOI: 10.1183/13993003.01378-2019

[105] Fujimoto K, Yasuo M, Urushibata K, et al. Airway inflammation during stable and acutely exacerbated chronic obstructive pulmonary disease. The European Respiratory Journal. 2005;**25**:640-646. DOI: 10.1183/09031936.05.00047504

[106] Leigh R, Pizzichini MM, Morris MM, et al. Stable COPD: Predicting benefit from high-dose inhaled corticosteroid treatment. The European Respiratory Journal. 2006;**27**:964-971. DOI: 10.1183/09031936.06.00072105

[107] Donohue JF, Betts KA, Du EX, et al. Comparative efficacy of long-acting β_2-agonists as monotherapy for chronic obstructive pulmonary disease: A network meta-analysis. International Journal of Chronic Obstructive Pulmonary Disease. 2017;**12**:367-381. DOI: 10.2147/COPD.S119908

[108] Rossi A, Centanni S, Cerveri I, et al. Acute effects of indacaterol on lung hyperinflation in moderate COPD: A comparison with tiotropium. Respiratory Medicine. 2012;**106**:84-90. DOI: 10.1016/j.rmed.2011.09.006

[109] Scherr A, Schafroth Török S, Jochmann A, et al. Response to add-on inhaled corticosteroids in COPD based

on airway hyperresponsiveness to mannitol. Chest. 2012;**142**:919-926. DOI: 10.1378/chest.11-2535

[110] Siddiqui SH, Pavord ID, Barnes NC, et al. Blood eosinophils: A biomarker of COPD exacerbation reduction with inhaled corticosteroids. International Journal of Chronic Obstructive Pulmonary Disease. 2018;**13**:3669-3676. DOI: 10.2147/COPD.S179425

[111] Kume H, Fukunaga K, Oguma T. Research and development of bronchodilators for asthma and COPD with a focus on G protein/K_{Ca} channel linkage and β_2-adrenergic intrinsic efficacy. Pharmacology & Therapeutics. 2015;**156**:75-89. DOI: 10.1016/j.pharmthera.2015.09.004

[112] Kume H, Ito S. Role of large-conductance calcium-activated potassium channels on airway smooth muscle in physiological and pathological conditions. In: Kume H, editor. Potassium Channels in Health and Disease. New York: Nova Science Publishers; 2017. pp. 41-120

[113] Kume H, Nishiyama O, Isoya T, et al. Involvement of allosteric effect and K_{Ca} channels in crosstalk between β-adrenergic and muscarinic M_2 receptors in airway smooth muscle. International Journal of Molecular Sciences. 2018;**19**:1999. DOI: 10.3390/ijms19071999

[114] Kume H. Research and development for anti-asthmatic agents with a focus on phenotype changing by Ca^{2+} signaling in airway smooth muscle cells. In: Rahman AU, editor. Frontiers in Clinical Drug Research - Anti Allergy Agents. Vol. 3. Sharjah, United Arab Emirates: Bentham; 2018. pp. 116-181

[115] Kume H. Role of airway smooth muscle in inflammation related to asthma and COPD. Advances in Experimental Medicine and Biology. 2018;**19**:1999

[116] Woodruff PG, Agusti A, Roche N, et al. Current concepts in targeting chronic obstructive pulmonary disease pharmacotherapy: Making progress towards personalised management. Lancet. 2015;**385**:1789-1798. DOI: 10.1016/S0140-6736(15)60693-6

[117] Washko GR, Parraga G. COPD biomarkers and phenotypes: Opportunities for better outcomes with precision imaging. The European Respiratory Journal. 2018;**52**:1801570. DOI: 10.1183/13993003.01570-2018

[118] Sidhaye VK, Nishida K, Martinez FJ. Precision medicine in COPD: Where are we and where do we need to go? European Respiratory Review. 2018;**27**:180022. DOI: 10.1183/16000617.0022-2018

[119] Brightling C, Greening N. Airway inflammation in COPD: Progress to precision medicine. The European Respiratory Journal. 2019;**54**:1900651. DOI: 10.1183/13993003.00651-2019

Chapter 8

Intratracheally Therapeutic Option for COPD: A Potential Usage of the Therapeutic Microbe for Delivering Specific Protein to the Lungs

Takashi Sato and Takeshi Shimosato

Abstract

Currently, inhaled therapy using corticosteroids and/or bronchodilators is the major established treatment for chronic obstructive pulmonary disease (COPD). The topic to be covered in this chapter is the recently developed experimental approach using biologically active molecules secreted by the live genetically modified lactic acid bacteria (gmLAB). The strategy to use gmLAB as a therapeutic/delivering tool targeting disease-specific active molecules/cites is proceeding. The role of inflammation and oxidative stress in COPD development is a valid target point. Heme oxygenase (HO)-1 as an anti-inflammatory and antioxidative stress molecule has been examined to attenuate the lung function decline and inflammation in the murine model of COPD. Recently, HO-1-secreting gmLAB as a tool for targeting inflammatory diseases has been developed and examined in several disease models including COPD. When administered intratracheally, the gmLAB showed migration to the peripheral lung and overexpression of anti-inflammatory/oxidative HO-1 in both lung and serum, protecting the lung from COPD development.

Keywords: chronic obstructive pulmonary disease, inhaled therapy, intratracheal therapy, anti-inflammatory therapy, antioxidative therapy, genetically modified lactic acid bacteria, heme oxygenase-1

1. Introduction

Chronic obstructive pulmonary disease (COPD) is characterized by airway remodeling due to chronic inflammation and subsequent airflow limitation that should be considered most to be associated with chronic symptoms such as shortness of breath and dyspnea [1]. Inhaled bronchodilators of long-acting beta-2 agonist/muscarinic antagonist have been introduced to treat symptomatic COPD [2]. Recently, more focus on the inflammation as a background condition of COPD is growing attention to a therapeutic factor to be considered [3]. In this regard, an inhaled corticosteroid (ICS) has been involved in the standard therapy for moderate to severe COPD. However, using ICS raises the concern of an increased risk of pneumonia [4]. Thus, another class of anti-inflammatory therapeutic options would be awaited. In line with this concept, experimental anti-inflammatory therapy using heme oxygenase (HO)-1 administration or induction in murine lung disease model including emphysema has been reported with successful amelioration of disease progression [5, 6]. HO catalyzes the degradation of heme to biliverdin, carbon monoxide (CO), and iron [7]. Thus, the by-products of biliverdin and CO act as anti-inflammatory and antioxidative agents [8, 9]. The results showing that the serum levels of HO-1 in patients with COPD having significantly lower compared to those in healthy adults could support the benefits of HO-1 adminitration/induction in the lungs of COPD [10]. A recent report indicates that the HO-1 could regulate lung inflammatory/oxidtative stress status by modulating mitogen-activated protein kinase (MAPK) pathway especially for extracellular signal-regulated kinase (ERK) [11].

There are several ways of induction and/or upregulation of HO-1 in the lungs by 1) chemical induction using hemin or CoPP [10, 12] and 2) local/systemic administration of recombinant HO-1 [5, 6, 13].

Especially, the use of generally recognized as safe (GRAS) materials such as lactic acid bacteria (LAB) for producing/delivering the therapeutics for human diseases such as inflammatory bowel disease and colorectal cancer has been gaining growing attention [14–17]. In addition, exploring the conceptional use of GRAS materials for lung diseases has been planned and tried for an experimental COPD model [13, 18].

This chapter summarizes the detailed experimental approach of the intratracheal administration of GRAS microbes for producing/delivering therapeutics in the COPD model.

2. Usage of lactic acid bacteria for intratracheal administration

2.1 Construction of genetically modified lactic acid bacteria (LAB)

There have been various LABs constructed for specific target therapy and/or monitoring the LAB dynamics after administration in the animal/human body. Lactococcus (L.) lactis NZ9000 for nisin regulated target gene expression system (MoBiTec, Goettingen, Germany) was used for these purposes. The genetically modified *L. lactis* was grown under the anaerobic condition at 30°C in M17 broth (BD Difico™) overnight. The target gene expression was induced by adding 1.25 ng/mL of nisin (MoBiTec). Of these gmLABs, a green fluorescent protein (GFP)-fusion target gene expressing LAB enables researchers to monitor the levels of target gene expressions [19]. **Figure 1** shows the vector constructed for monitoring the time-dependent migration after nasally administering *Lactococcus lactis* that express/produce GFP over time.

The GFP-expressing *L. lactis* was cultured, and further time course was monitored for expression levels of GFP. Three hours after adding nisin (1.25 ng/mL), the cultured/induced GFP-expressing *L. lactis* was visualized under fluorescent microscope observation (**Figure 2**).

2.2 Airway migration of nasally administered *L. lactis*

GFP-expressing *L. lactis* were nasally administered to the anesthetized mice. A total of 50 μL of saline containing 1.0×10^9 of *L. lactis* was dropped into the nares and migrated to the lungs through stable nasal breathing.

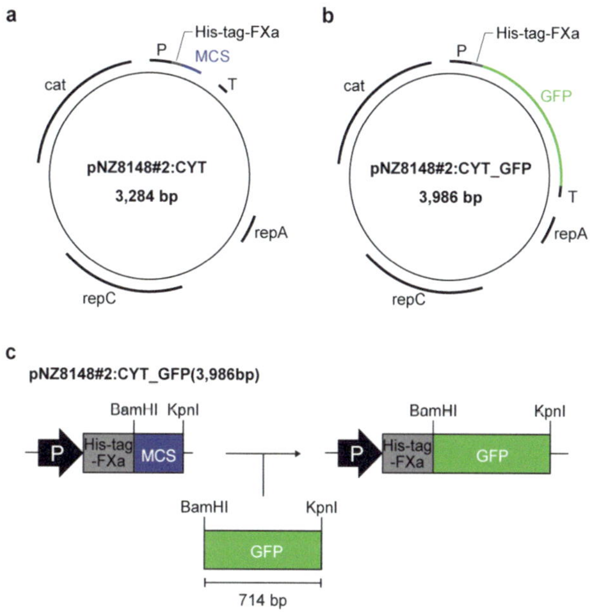

Figure 1.
Construction of GFP-expressing vector incorporated into the LAB. (a) lactococcal plasmid pNZ8148#2:CYT. (b) A green fluorescent protein (GFP) expression vector (pNZ8148#2:CYT_GFP). (c) Vector map of the pNZ8148#2:CYT_GFP. Notes: P = nisin A promotor; His-tag = hexahistidine tag; FXa = Factor Xa recognition site; MCS = multiple cloning site; T = terminator; rep = replication gene; and cat = chloramphenicol acetyltrasferase gene.

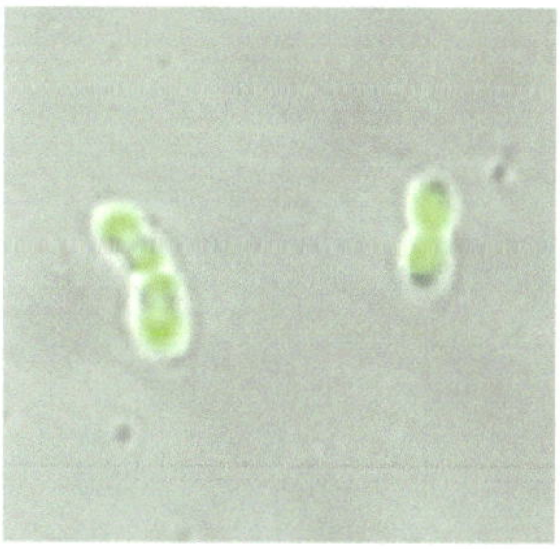

Figure 2.
Image of GFP-expressing Lactococcus lactis after induction with nisin. Genetically modified Lactococcus (L.) lactis were cultured and further induced with nisin for expression of a specific protein. The high-power field image of L. lactis showing diplococci morphology with a green signal derived from the GFP expression vector-incorporated system was visualized using a fluorescent microscope (BZ-X800; Keyence, Japan).

As shown in **Figure 3**, visualized GFP signal was time-dependently moved from the central lesion to the peripheral lesion of the lungs. Finally, the GFP signal was cleared from the lungs 96 after administration. Notably, at the same time of 96 hr, there was still an apparent GFP signal in the trachea, indicating 1) the high affinity of *L. lactis* for tracheal epithelium and 2) the potential usage of *L. lactis* as a carrier of airway mucosal vaccination.

2.3 Systemic effect of nasally administered *L. lactis*

Potential systemic influences after administering *L. lactis* would be body temperature, body weight, and eating behavior. Of these, time-course analysis of percent

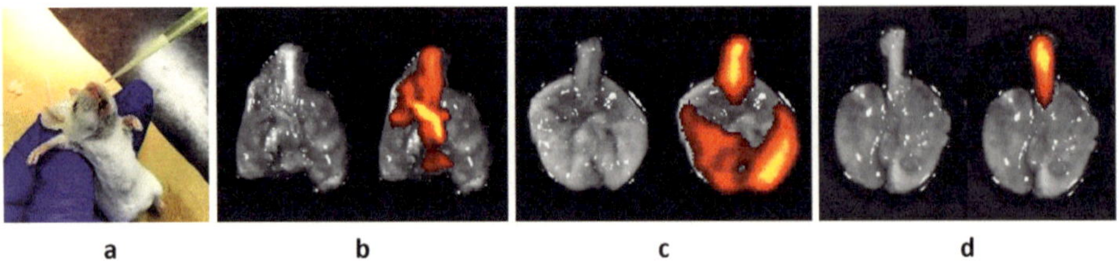

Figure 3.
Time-course analysis of ex vivo fluorescence images of removed lungs after administering GFP-expressing L. lactis. *(a) Mice (8–9 weeks of age) administered nasally with 1.0 × 10^9 of GFP-expressing* L. lactis *under anesthetized with pentobarbital sodium (30 mg/kg) were euthanized at an indicated timepoint of (b) 24 hr, (c) 48 hr, and (d) 96 hr. The removed lungs were observed under IVIS (In Vivo Imaging System, Perkin-Elmer) with (right panel) or without (left panel) fluorescence excitation. GFP signal visualized in right panel at each time point appeared in the central lesion (trachea and hilar area of the lungs) at 24 hr (b), moved to the peripheral lesion at 48 hr (c), and cleared from the lungs at 96 hr (d).*

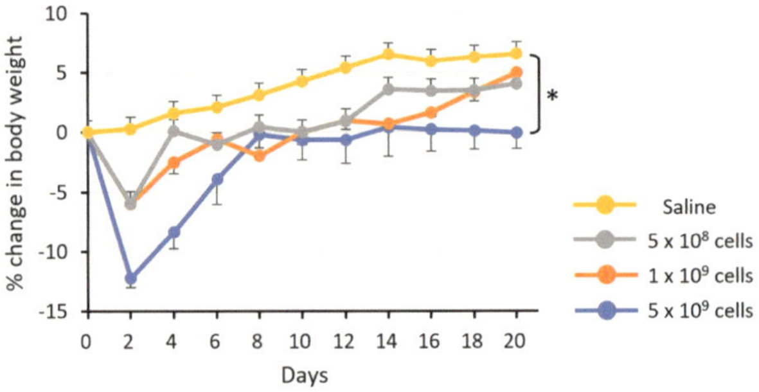

Figure 4.
Change in body weight after nasal administration of L. lactis. Time-course analysis of percent change in body weight in mice (8–9 weeks of age) administered nasally with 0, 5 × 10^8, 1 × 10^9, or 5 × 10^9 of L. lactis. Results showed that a significant body weight loss was observed in mice treated with 5 × 10^9 of L. lactis. The calculated area under the curve of body weight from 3 to 4 mice per group indicated a statistically significant body weight loss in 5 × 10^9 of the L. lactis group compared with the saline group. $^*p < 0.05$. *Adapted from reference [13].*

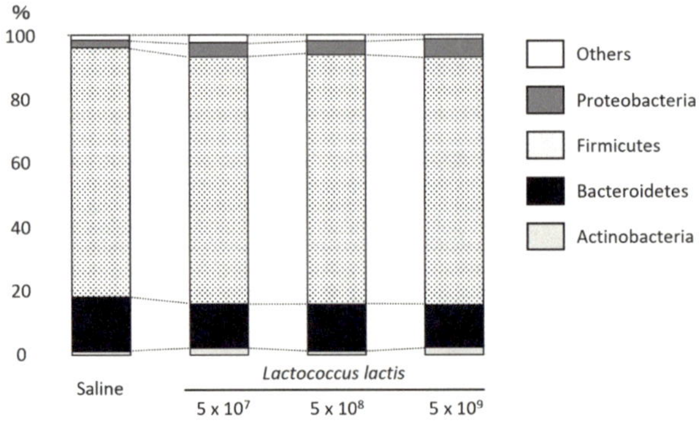

Figure 5.
Analysis of lung microbiota 14 days after nasal administration of L. lactis. Mice (8–9 weeks of age) administered nasally with 0, 5 × 10^7, 5 × 10^8, or 5 × 10^9 of L. lactis were euthanized and collected bronchoalveolar lavage (BAL) fluids 14 days after administration. The analysis of the 16S rRNA gene (V3-V4 region) was amplified and subjected to next-generation sequencing (3 mice per group).

change in body weight showed the safety concern of mice (8–9 weeks of age) administered nasally with over 1 × 10^9 of *L. lactis*. As shown in **Figure 4**, the calculated area under the curve of body weight from 3 to 4 mice per group indicated a statistically significant body weight loss in 5 × 10^9 of the *L. lactis* group compared with the saline group. Based on these results, the optimized amount of nasal administration of *L. lactis* was set to less than 1 × 10^9 per body at one time.

2.4 Local effects of nasally administered *L. lactis*

Another concern after nasally administering *L. lactis* would be a potential alteration of lung microbiota. As shown in **Figure 5**, intratracheal administration of up to 5 × 10^9 of *L. lactis* would show no statistical significance in 1) Bacteroidetes to Firmicutes ratio and 2) the composition of the microbiota belonging to Bacteroidetes or Firmicutes compared with those observed in control (saline) group.

3. Usage of lactic acid bacteria for COPD model

3.1 Construction of genetically modified *L. lactis* secreting anti-inflammatory/antioxidative stress protein HO-1

To explore the anti-inflammatory therapeutic option other than corticosteroids in COPD, HO-1 was focused on because of its low serum level shown in patients with COPD [10]. The newly constructed HO-1 secreting *L. lactis* (**Figure 6**) was examined by oral administration in a dextran sulfate sodium-induced murine colitis model [17]. Since the favorable alleviation of disease symptoms was observed in this model, a further trial was planned for lung diseases by exploring another delivery method of intratracheal administration. **Figure 6** shows the vector constructed for the HO-1 secreting *L. lactis* NZ9000 system.

3.2 HO-1 production in the lungs after nasally administering HO-1 *L. lactis*

HO-1 secreting *L. lactis* were nasally administered to the anesthetized mice. A total of 50 μL of saline containing 1.0 × 10^9 of *L. lactis* was migrated to the lungs through stable nasal breathing. Production of HO-1 derived from HO-1 *L. lactis* was confirmed by immunoblotting using anti-His antibody and anti-HO-1 antibody in lung homogenates (**Figure 7a**). Through the pulmonary trafficking of HO-1 *L. lactis*, serum HO-1 levels were significantly increased (**Figure 7b**).

3.3 Effect of nasally administered HO-1 secreting *L. lactis* in murine emphysema model

HO-1-secreting *L. lactis* were nasally administered to the anesthetized mice 48 hr before instillation with porcine pancreatic elastase (PPE) (**Figure 8**). A total of 50 μL of saline containing 1.0 × 10^9 of *L. lactis* was dropped into the nares and migrated to the lungs through stable nasal breathing.

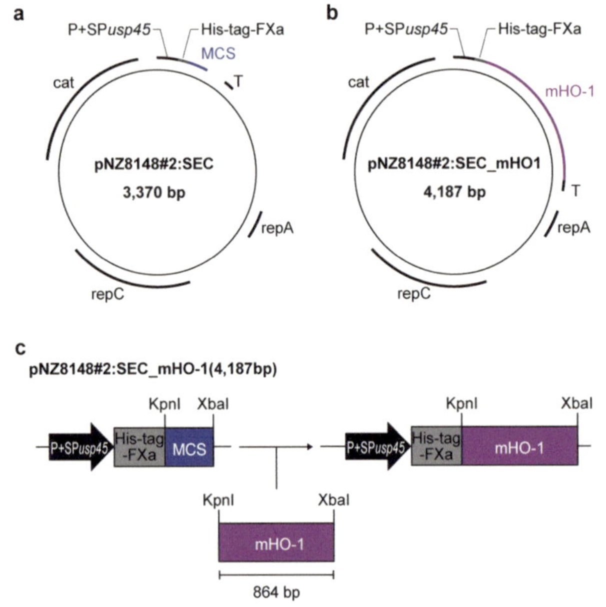

Figure 6.
Construction of HO-1-expressing vector incorporated into L. lactis. (a) A lactococcal plasmid pNZ8148#2:SEC. (b) A heme oxygenase-1 (HO-1) expression vector (pNZ8148#2:SEC_mHO1). (c) Vector map of the pNZ8148#2:SEC_mHO1. Notes: P = nisin A promotor; SP_{USP45} = sequence of the signal peptide from the USP45 protein; His-tag = hexahistidine tag; FXa = Factor Xa recognition site; MCS = multiple cloning site; T = terminator; rep = replication gene; and cat = chloramphenicol acetyltrasferase gene.

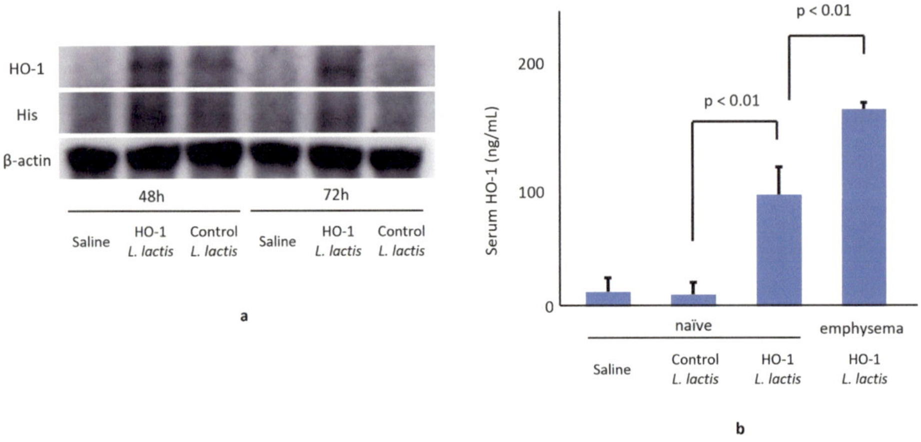

Figure 7.
Systemic and local HO-1 production after nasal administration of HO-1 L. lactis. Mice (8–9 weeks of age) administered nasally with HO-1 L. lactis were subjected to assess the local (lung) and systemic (serum) HO-1 levels 48 or 72 hr after administration. (a) The lung homogenates from naïve mice receiving either control or HO-1 L. lactis were assessed by immunoblotting. The representative result showed that the nisin-induced HO-1 was confirmed. Adapted from reference [13]. (b) Serum HO-1 levels were assessed using ELISA (MK125, TAKARA Bio Inc., Japan) 48 hr after administration. Results from 5 to 6 mice/group showed a significant increase in HO-1 in both naïve and emphysema models receiving HO-1 L. lactis compared with those receiving control L. lactis.

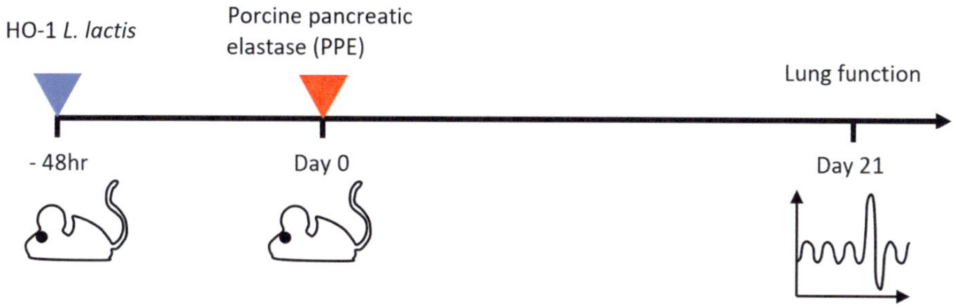

Figure 8.
Protocol of the prophylactic use of HO-1 L. lactis in emphysema model. HO-1 L. lactis was administered 48 hr before instillation of 1 unit of porcine pancreatic elastase (PPE; Elastin Products Co., Inc., USA) in 50 μL of saline. The mice treated with PPE showed progressive destruction of the alveolar structure, leading to emphysematous morphologic deterioration up to day 21.

On day 21, after PPE instillation, the mice developing pulmonary emphysema were evaluated by pulmonary function test using the flexiVent system (emka TECHNOLOGIES Japan).

3.3.1 Systemic effect of nasally administered HO-1 secreting L. lactis

Mice pretreated with 1.0×10^9 of HO-1 *L. lactis* showed a significant increase in body weight compared with those pretreated with control *L. lactis* or only saline

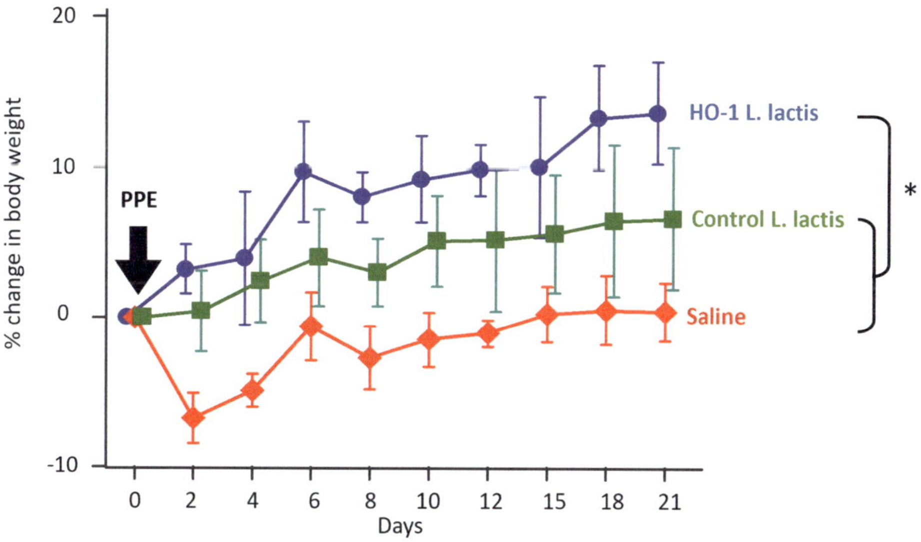

Figure 9.
*Effect of nasal administration of L. lactis on PPE-induced weight loss. Time-course analysis of percent change in body weight after PPE instillation (Day 0) in mice pretreated nasally with 1×10^9 of either HO-1 L. lactis or control L. lactis (Day -2). A significant body weight loss observed in mice pretreated with saline (vehicle only) was not reproduced in mice pretreated with HO-1 L. lactis. The calculated area under the curve of body weight from 5 to 6 mice per group indicated a statistically significant improvement in body weight loss in the HO-1 L. lactis group compared with the control L. lactis or saline group. * $p < 0.05$. Adapted from reference [13].*

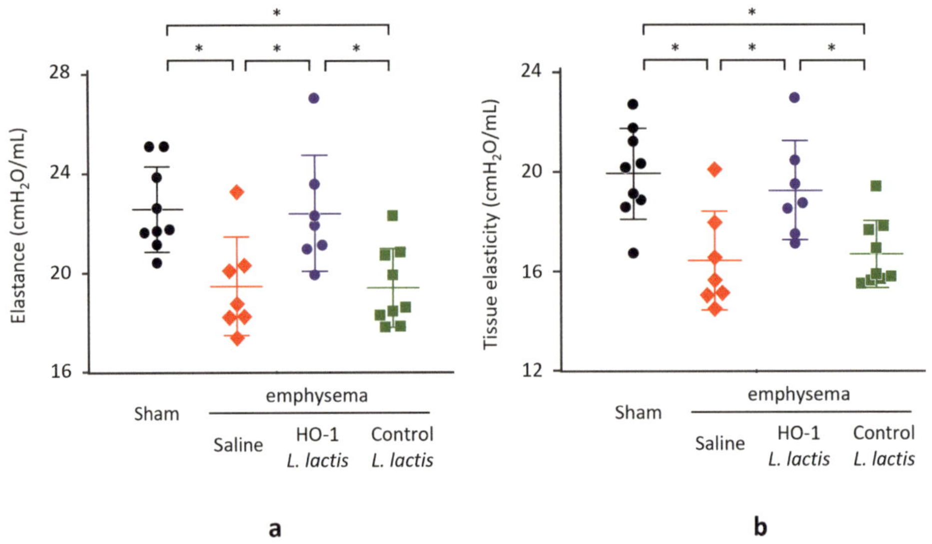

Figure 10.
*Local effect of nasally administered HO-1 L. lactis on PPE-induced emphysema mice assessed by in vivo lung function measurements. Mice were treated as described in **Figure 8**. In vivo lung function tests were performed under anesthesia using a flexiVent system on day 21. The results of lung function measurements of (a) Elastance and (b) Tissue elasticity were shown. Bars indicate the mean ± SD. * $p < 0.05$. Adapted from reference [13].*

($p < 0.05$) (**Figure 9**). Thus, nasal administration of HO-1 *L. lactis* reduced the physiological deterioration caused by PPE.

3.3.2 Local effect of nasally administered HO-1 secreting L. lactis

In human clinical trials, the efficacy of candidate drugs for COPD should be primarily assessed by inhibiting lung function deterioration [20]. Therefore, in vivo lung function measurements of mice receiving with or without HO-1 *L. lactis* before emphysema development were assessed using a highly sensitive and reproducible flexiVent system for small animal [21]. The characteristic of an emphysematous lung is reduced elasticity reflecting the hyperinflation and decreased elastic recoil [21]. Consistent with this lung morphologic deterioration, "elastance" (determined by single-frequency forced oscillation technique) and "tissue elasticity" (defined by a small amplitude broadband oscillation technique) were significantly decreased in PPE-induced emphysema mice pretreated with either saline or control *L. lactis*. Fortunately, however, the mice pretreated with HO-1 *L. lactis* showed satisfactory suppression of PPE-induced lung function deterioration (**Figure 10**).

4. Conclusions

This chapter summarizes the potential therapeutics of gmLAB and its application for lung diseases, including COPD. LAB has been widely used as probiotics for health, and to maximize its beneficial effects, gmLAB has been developed. Among several gmLABs, the use of *L. lactis* has been favored because of 1) its generally recognized as safe status, 2) its absence of endotoxins, 3) its easy manipulating property, and 4) its low cost and easy administration. When applied for lung diseases, direct delivery of the therapeutics (gmLAB) to the lungs by intratracheal administration would be favored in terms of efficacy and safety concerns. In addition, the successful attenuation of disease progression in the murine emphysema model by local administration of anti-inflammatory gmLAB would support a further human clinical trial.

Acknowledgements

Authors thank Drs. Kentaro Nakashima and Kentaro Yumoto (Yokohama City University, Japan) and Drs. Suguru Shigemori and Fu Namai (Shinshu University, Japan) for their significant contribution to the project. The project was funded by the Japan Society for the Promotion of Science (JSPS) KAKENHI, grant numbers JP15K09224, JP18K19935, JP19KK0208, and JP22K08578 to Takashi Sato.

Conflict of interest

The authors declare no conflict of interest.

Author details

Takashi Sato* and Takeshi Shimosato
Institute for Biomedical Sciences, Shinshu University, Nagano, Japan

*Address all correspondence to: satotak@shinshu-u.ac.jp

References

[1] James AL, Wenzel S. Clinical relevance of airway remodelling in airway diseases. The European Respiratory Journal. 2007;**30**(1):134-155. DOI: 10.1183/09031936.00146905

[2] Page C, Cazzola M. Bifunctional drugs for the treatment of asthma and chronic obstructive pulmonary disease. The European Respiratory Journal. 2014;**44**(2):475-482. DOI: 10.1183/09031936.00003814

[3] King PT. Inflammation in chronic obstructive pulmonary disease and its role in cardiovascular disease and lung cancer. Clinical and Translational Medicine. 2015;**4**(1):68. DOI: 10.1186/s40169-015-0068-z

[4] Wang CY, Lai CC, Yang WC, Lin CC, Chen L, Wang HC, et al. The association between inhaled corticosteroid and pneumonia in COPD patients: The improvement of patients' life quality with COPD in Taiwan (IMPACT) study. International Journal of Chronic Obstructive Pulmonary Disease. 2016;**11**:2775-2783. DOI: 10.2147/COPD.S116750

[5] Otterbein LE, Kolls JK, Mantell LL, Cook JL, Alam J, Choi AM. Exogenous administration of heme oxygenase-1 by gene transfer provides protection against hyperoxia-induced lung injury. The Journal of Clinical Investigation. 1999;**103**(7):1047-1054. DOI: 10.1172/JCI5342

[6] Shinohara T, Kaneko T, Nagashima Y, Ueda A, Tagawa A, Ishigatsubo Y. Adenovirus-mediated transfer and overexpression of heme oxygenase 1 cDNA in lungs attenuates elastase-induced pulmonary emphysema in mice. Human Gene Therapy. 2005;**16**(3):318-327. DOI: 10.1089/hum.2005.16.318

[7] Tenhunen R, Marver HS, Schmid R. The enzymatic conversion of heme to bilirubin by microsomal heme oxygenase. Proceedings of the National Academy of Sciences of the United States of America. 1968;**61**(2):748-755. DOI: 10.1073/pnas.61.2.748

[8] Otterbein LE, Bach FH, Alam J, Soares M, Tao Lu H, Wysk M, et al. Carbon monoxide has anti-inflammatory effects involving the mitogen-activated protein kinase pathway. Nature Medicine. 2000;**6**(4):422-428. DOI: 10.1038/74680

[9] Stocker R, Yamamoto Y, McDonagh AF, Glazer AN, Ames BN. Bilirubin is an antioxidant of possible physiological importance. Science. 1987;**235**(4792):1043-1046. DOI: 10.1126/science.3029864

[10] Sato T, Takeno M, Honma K, Yamauchi H, Saito Y, Sasaki T, et al. Heme oxygenase-1, a potential biomarker of chronic silicosis, attenuates silica-induced lung injury. American Journal of Respiratory and Critical Care Medicine. 2006;**174**(8):906-914. DOI: 10.1164/rccm.200508-1237OC

[11] Nakashima K, Sato T, Shigemori S, Shimosato T, Shinkai M, Kaneko T. Regulatory role of heme oxygenase-1 in silica-induced lung injury. Respiratory Research. 2018;**19**(1):144. DOI: 10.1186/s12931-018-0852-6

[12] Minamoto K, Harada H, Lama VN, Fedarau MA, Pinsky DJ. Reciprocal regulation of airway rejection by the inducible gas-forming enzymes heme oxygenase and nitric oxide synthase.

The Journal of Experimental Medicine. 2005;**202**(2):283-294. DOI: 10.1084/jem.20050377

[13] Yumoto K, Sato T, Nakashima K, Namai F, Shigemori S, Shimosato T, et al. Nasally administered lactococcus lactis secreting heme oxygenase-1 attenuates murine emphysema. Antioxidants (Basel). 2020;**9**(11): 283-294. DOI: 10.3390/antiox9111049

[14] Ciacma K, Wieckiewicz J, Kedracka-Krok S, Kurtyka M, Stec M, Siedlar M, et al. Secretion of tumoricidal human tumor necrosis factor-related apoptosis-inducing ligand (TRAIL) by recombinant Lactococcus lactis: Optimization of in vitro synthesis conditions. Microbial Cell Factories. 2018;**17**(1):177. DOI: 10.1186/s12934-018-1028-2

[15] Namai F, Shigemori S, Ogita T, Sato T, Shimosato T. Microbial therapeutics for acute colitis based on genetically modified Lactococcus lactis hypersecreting IL-1Ra in mice. Experimental & Molecular Medicine. 2020;**52**(9):1627-1636. DOI: 10.1038/s12276-020-00507-5

[16] Shigemori S, Shimosato T. Applications of genetically modified immunobiotics with high immunoregulatory capacity for treatment of inflammatory bowel diseases. Frontiers in Immunology. 2017;**8**:22. DOI: 10.3389/fimmu.2017.00022

[17] Shigemori S, Watanabe T, Kudoh K, Ihara M, Nigar S, Yamamoto Y, et al. Oral delivery of Lactococcus lactis that secretes bioactive heme oxygenase-1 alleviates development of acute colitis in mice. Microbial Cell Factories. 2015;**14**:189. DOI: 10.1186/s12934-015-0378-2

[18] Sato T, Shimosato T. Development of a New Treatment Modality for Lung Diseases That Uses Innovative Fine Droplet Drying (fdd) Technology Offering Inhalable Nano/microparticles-incorporated Therapeutic Agents. New York: Science Impact Ltd; 2019. DOI: 10.21820/23987073.2019.3.56

[19] Shigemori S, Namai F, Yamamoto Y, Nigar S, Sato T, Ogita T, et al. Genetically modified Lactococcus lactis producing a green fluorescent protein-bovine lactoferrin fusion protein suppresses proinflammatory cytokine expression in lipopolysaccharide-stimulated RAW 264.7 cells. Journal of Dairy Science. 2017;**100**(9):7007-7015. DOI: 10.3168/jds.2017-12872

[20] Cazzola M, MacNee W, Martinez FJ, Rabe KF, Franciosi LG, Barnes PJ, et al. Outcomes for COPD pharmacological trials: From lung function to biomarkers. The European Respiratory Journal. 2008;**31**(2):416-469. DOI: 10.1183/09031936.00099306

[21] Vanoirbeek JA, Rinaldi M, De Vooght V, Haenen S, Bobic S, Gayan-Ramirez G, et al. Noninvasive and invasive pulmonary function in mouse models of obstructive and restrictive respiratory diseases. American Journal of Respiratory Cell and Molecular Biology. 2010;**42**(1):96-104. DOI: 10.1165/rcmb.2008-0487OC